massage

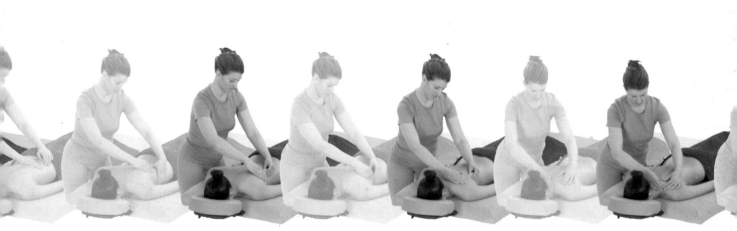

a *flowmotion*™ title

massage

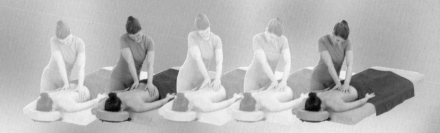

rosie linda harness
& nuro weidemann

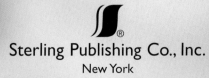

Sterling Publishing Co., Inc.
New York

Created and conceived by
Axis Publishing Limited
8c Accommodation Road
London NW11 8ED
www.axispublishing.co.uk

Creative Director: Siân Keogh
Editorial Director: Brian Burns
Project Designer: Axis Design Editions
Managing Editor: Conor Kilgallon
Production Manager: Tim Clarke
Photographer: Mike Good

Library of Congress Cataloging-in-Publication Data
Available

10 9 8 7 6 5 4 3 2 1

Published in 2003 by Sterling Publishing Co., Inc.
387 Park Avenue South, New York, NY 10016
Text and images © Axis Publishing Limited 2003
Distributed in Canada by Sterling Publishing
C/o Canadian Manda Group,
One Atlantic Avenue, Suite 105
Toronto, Ontario, Canada, M6K 3E7

ISBN 1–4027–0903–X

Printed by Star Standard (Pte) Limited

The publishers would like to thank Majestic Towels
Ltd, Birmingham, UK, for providing the towels, and the
Massage Table Store, London, UK, for providing the
massage chair and table.

For more information on holistic massage, contact
the College of Holistic Massage UK (info@chmuk.net)
or visit www.chmuk.net

a *flow**motion*™ title

massage

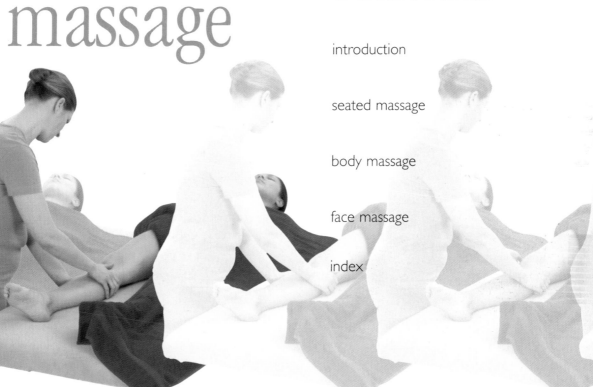

contents

introduction

Touch, one of our deepest instinctual responses, is as old as the ages and as immediate as this moment. It can convey the subtlest shades of expression through the widest range of feelings. A mother's natural impulse to kiss, rub, or stroke a hurt child appears to bring an almost magical and instant soothing. Our instinct to reach out to touch and comfort a person in need arises from a place beyond the rational mind. And when, in massage, touch is conveyed with intention, respect, caring, and expertise, the effect can be profoundly soothing and balancing for the body, mind, emotions, and soul.

Massage is now beginning to claim its rightful place, not only among the wide range of alternative body therapies, but also within the medical profession. Recognition is coming that massage is a valid therapy—one that can provide relief for aches and pains, release stress and tension, promote relaxation, and, because of these attributes, be an invaluable preventive medicine.

history

Although it may seem that massage is just being discovered, it existed as a form of healing at least 5,000 years ago, in China, Japan, and India. In 3000 B.C., some of the earliest Chinese medical writings mention that "early morning effleurage with the palm of the hand, after a night's sleep when the blood is rested and the temper more relaxed, protects against cold,

Massage is not a luxury for the rich or an indulgence of mellow sensualists. . . it is a vital rhythmic interplay that should be part of everybody's life.

(GABRIELLE ROTH, MAPS TO ECSTASY)

keeps the organs supple, and prevents many minor ailments." Around the same time, Hindu priests were writing that "massage reduces fat, strengthens the muscles and firms the skin."

A wall painting from an Egyptian tomb in 2330 B.C. clearly shows practitioners giving foot and hand massage to their clients, and an illustration from the Canon of Avicenna (A.D. 980–1037) shows a vigorous back massage being performed. The art of massage, far from being just a tool for pampering, was used by the ancient Greek and Roman physicians as one of the principal ways of relieving pain. In the year 380 B.C., Hippocrates, the "father of medicine," wrote that "a physician must be experienced in many things, but assuredly also in rubbing." The Greeks prescribed massage for their patients as well as for their athletes.

The Roman Empire enthusiastically adopted these practices. Galen informs us in the 2nd century A.D. that "massage eliminates the waste

THE BENEFITS OF MASSAGE

physical:

- Improves skin tone and color by removing dead cells
- Improves blood circulation which provides a more efficient delivery of nutrients and oxygen to cells and more efficient waste removal
- Encourages deeper, and therefore more efficient and relaxed, breathing
- Relieves muscle fatigue, stiffness, and soreness
- Can counteract insomnia
- Boosts the immune system
- Helps release energy blocks and redistributes and balances the body's energy

psychological:

- Relaxes the body, reducing tension and the effects of stress
- Relaxes the mind, thereby reducing anxiety and its effects
- Soothes and comforts
- Increases general vitality and a feeling of well-being by invigorating all the body's systems
- Improves body awareness and self-esteem

spiritual:

- Helps to integrate body, mind, and spirit into a more harmonious balance, offering an opportunity to reconnect with the essential self and to view life from a different perspective
- Provides valuable time and space in a pressurized world to return to a state of "being" rather than "doing."

products of nutrition and the poisons of fatigue." After the fall of Rome in the 5th century, the importance of massage as a healing tool declined. It resurfaced in the 11th century when Avicenna, an Arab philosopher and physician, noted that the object of massage was to "disperse the effete matters found in the muscles and not expelled by exercise."

It is unlikely that something as important and as basic as massage disappeared completely, but it did appear to go underground in the Middle Ages, reappearing in the 16th century through the work and writings of a French doctor, Ambrose Pare. In the early 19th century, a Swede, Per Henrik Ling, cured himself of rheumatism by synthesizing a system of massage through his knowledge of gymnastics and physiology and Chinese, Egyptian, Greek, and Roman massage techniques. And it is from this form of Swedish massage that most soft-tissue intuitive and holistic massage has evolved.

Place a small amount of oil in the palm of your hand to begin. Add more later if necessary.

key elements of massage

quality of touch

The quality of the touch you bring to a massage is as important as your technique. Try this exercise to help you experience "touch" in an immediate way: Sit quietly where you will not be disturbed. Think of someone you love and let that feeling flow down to your hands. Then, slowly place your hands on your face as lovingly as you would touch the person you love. Let the whole of your hand envelop the contours of your face and allow yourself to really feel the quality of the touch, its softness, caring, and the way these feelings are conveyed. Spend some time covering all parts of your face and head in this way, allowing yourself to receive your own loving touch. These are the qualities to bring to your massage.

conveying intention

Intention, focus, and presence are also vital ingredients in a good massage. To get in touch with these and get a taste of what you will be conveying to your partner, try this:

Sit comfortably with your eyes closed. Become aware of your breath, and as you inhale, bring your breath into your heart area (mid-chest); as you exhale, imagine the energy from your breath flowing out of your arms and hands, with the focus being the middle of your palms. Do this for five minutes, then bring your palms together, about ½in (1cm) apart. Focus on whatever the feeling is between the palms of your hands and try to describe to yourself as precisely as possible the sensation you experience. It is this energy and the connection between your palms that you need to bring to the massage and convey to your partner.

massage chair

The specially designed chair pictured here is ideal for supporting your partner comfortably while you work, but an acceptable alternative is a kitchen chair on which your partner can sit or straddle. This gives more accessibility when massaging the back.

massage couch
A massage couch is ideal for ease and comfort when working on your partner. It will fold in two for easy storage and transport.

WATCHWORDS

flow—Keep your strokes and movements smooth, flowing, and connected when moving from one part of the massage sequence to the other, without break or disruption.

feedback—Encourage your partner to give helpful or useful feedback such as "too deep" or "too light," but otherwise conduct the massage in silence; this will enable you and your partner to share a deeper experience.

giving—Give yourself time to learn massage, taking one sequence at a time. Being aware of posture, breath, centering, and grounding will help you relax and enjoy the process. Once you have mastered the strokes and sequences you can allow your intuition to play a larger part; you may then find your hands devising their own movements and strokes more suitable and appropriate for the needs of the person you are massaging.

receiving—If you are receiving a massage, allow yourself to relax as deeply as possible. Let your attention rest lightly on your breathing and give yourself up to the movement of the massage and the enjoyment of the experience.

grounding, centering, posture, and breathing

Intention, focus, and presence are supported by grounding, centering, good posture, and correct breathing. Grounding means that you are aware of your feet being in contact and connected with the ground. Keeping your knees slightly bent and flexible means that energy can flow up and down your legs, which it cannot do if your knees are locked.

Centering means that your focus and center of gravity come from the energy center (sometimes called a chakra) just below the navel. Think of a Hawaiian dancer and how the movement and strength comes from the lower half of the body, the hips, pelvis and legs.

Good posture is vital to a good massage—and the degree of comfort you experience in your body as you massage will be conveyed to your partner. A straight back, strong, flexible well-placed legs to support your body, and strong arms (not collapsed at the elbows) mean that you can use your body weight rather than your hands to do the work.

Deep breathing from the abdomen (rather than the chest) is calming and centering and it is important that you stay in touch with your breathing as you massage.

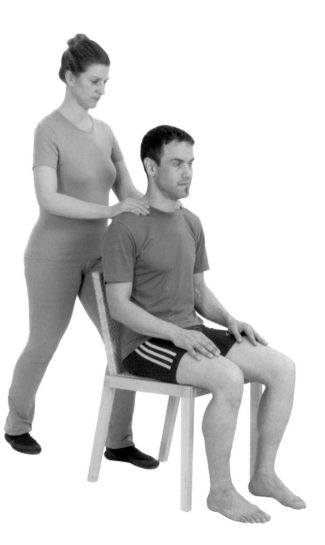

Good posture and technique are essential to a good massage, whether using a massage couch or a simple kitchen chair.

preparation

The more you can relax and center yourself before giving a massage, the more successful and effective the experience will be for you and your partner. Choose a way of preparing that suits you. This may be sitting quietly for 15 minutes, becoming aware of your breath, and allowing thoughts simply to come and go. Alternatively, you may like to dance around your living room to release the day's stresses, bringing your attention back to the rhythm any time your mind wanders. Or perhaps just the process of preparing a beautiful space for the massage to take place in may be relaxing and centering. Stretching and deep breathing can also help to center and ground the body and mind. What is important is to set aside some time and space for yourself before you begin the massage.

personal preparation

Because of the close proximity between you and your partner, special care needs to be taken with personal hygiene. Make sure you are freshly showered, have no strong flavors on your breath, use deodorant, and wear clean, light, comfortable clothes—a T-shirt, loose pants, and flat-soled shoes are ideal. Fingernails should be short and clean, and long hair tied back.

the right environment

Choose a peaceful room or space away from noise and distractions. It should be clean, ventilated, and very warm. Light some candles to provide a soft, warm glow and perhaps burn an essential oil to release a delicate fragrance.

For the massage, almond or grapeseed oils are ideal, either in a dispenser or small bowl. Unless you have a qualification in aromatherapy, it is best not to add essential oils to the massage oil, but excellent premixed oils that can enhance sensual massage, lift or relax the mood, and ease aching muscles are readily available in good drugstores and health food stores. Warming the massage oil makes a delicious addition to the massage.

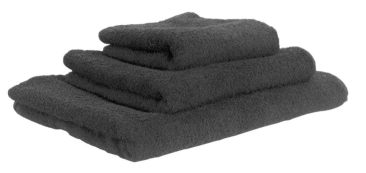

CORRECT BODY POSITION FOR FLOOR WORK

working parallel

When massaging from the floor, it is important to maintain a comfortable and easy posture. When working parallel to your partner (for example, with effleurage), face toward your partner's head with your right knee on the floor and lower leg parallel to the body. Have your left leg bent at the knee to provide stability and flexibility and keep your back straight to avoid collapsing at the waist. This way of working will become easy with practice.

working across the body (right and far right)

When working across the body (cupping, hacking, kneading, and so on), kneel with your right knee on the floor and your left knee raised to stabilize and support your arms. Reaching (not leaning) across your partner from the shoulders, with slightly rounded arms and straight back (not collapsed from the waist), will make this a comfortable position from which to work.

Soothing, quiet music can enhance the massage experience but your partner may prefer silence, so ask first. A vase of flowers or attractive plant may complete the scene.

Ideally, use a massage couch for physical ease and comfort. To find the ideal height, stand facing the couch with your knees slightly bent and your fists clenched. Your fist should clear the top of the table when swung backward and forward. Provide three clean and fluffy towels (two large, one small). One should be used to cover the couch and the other, already warmed, should be large enough to cover the whole of your partner's body, including the feet. The third (small) towel should be used to cover the breast area. If you have to work on the floor, create a comfortable and soft place to work, with extra padding under your knees and ankles, and avoid any drafts. Use the same principles of grounding, centering, posture, and breathing, but adapt to working on the floor.

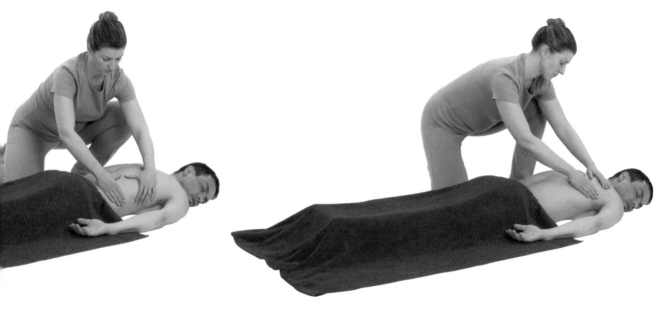

DO'S AND DON'TS (CONTRAINDICATIONS TO MASSAGE)

Massage has many beneficial effects on health and well-being. However, there are occasions when massage should be avoided or when medical advice is needed. You should never massage a pregnant woman. Avoid the following areas on a person's body:

- An infectious area of skin
- Varicose veins
- Inflamed joints

Do not massage anyone with:

- Heart problems
- Phlebitis
- Cancer or tumors
- Thrombosis
- Hypertension (high blood pressure)
- A fever

Always check beforehand whether the person to be massaged has any allergies or skin conditions that are sensitive to particular lotions, oils, or perfumes.

how massage works

Because the veins carry blood back to the heart, and lymph flows toward the major lymph vessels in the upper body, most strokes are performed toward the heart, to aid these processes. Therefore, generally, strokes are given a heavier emphasis as you massage up toward the heart and a lighter pressure on the downward journey. Massage is conducted in a rhythmic, flowing motion with as little disconnection as possible.

Think of massage as consisting of six sections, in the following order:

First: The back, working from the buttocks and lower back to the upper back and shoulders

Second: The backs of the legs, working from the feet to the upper thighs

Third: The shoulders, neck, and head (the face is optional)

Fourth: The abdomen and chest

Fifth: The arms

Sixth: The front of the legs, from feet to upper thighs

essential strokes

Massage includes a series of different and uniquely effective strokes that are used in each sequence. We recommend that you learn and practice the strokes first, and when you feel confident, begin the massage, starting with the back massage sequence. Practice each sequence until you are confident enough to move on to the next.

Holds: Holds are passive and are performed by placing your hands on different areas of the body, thereby creating an energy flow and connection between your hands and the recipient's body. Holds provide the opportunity for stillness, connection, and integration. Common holds are the sacrum and the back of the neck; a hand on each foot; connecting joints, such as the hip and ankle; and either side of the head.

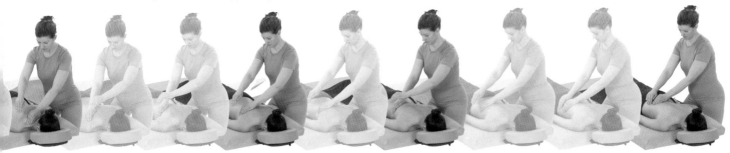

effleurage (stroking)

Effleurage derives from the French word *effleur*, to touch lightly.

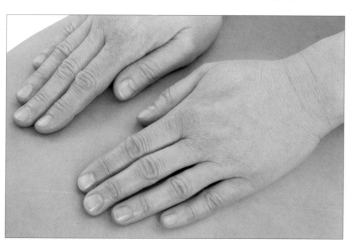

Soft knuckle stroke (right):
This slightly deeper effleurage stroke is used to stretch and lengthen large muscle areas and promote tension release and elasticity by stretching the muscle fibers.

Action: Form a loose fist, with your thumb acting as a pivot to stabilize the stroke. With the flat "soft" part of the knuckles, work into the muscle with a deep circular motion.

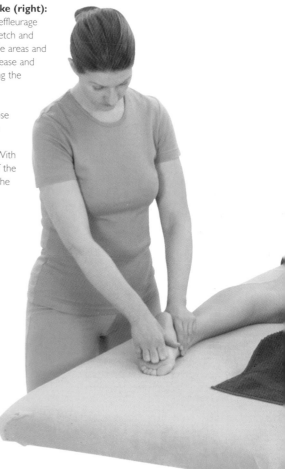

Effleurage (above): This is a gentle, sweeping, relaxing stroke with varying levels of pressure. Effleurage is used at the beginning and end of a sequence and to connect different massage strokes with one another. It familiarizes the receiver with the touch of the practitioner, soothes and relaxes the muscles, improves circulation, and induces a sense of deep relaxation. It also passively stretches and warms the muscles prior to deeper movements.

Action: Hold your fingers and thumbs together, keeping your hand relaxed, in contact with, and flowing over the contours of the body in long, slow, rhythmic movements. The emphasis and pressure occurs on the upward movement.

petrissage

Petrissage derives from the French word *pétrir*, which means to knead or rub with force, and uses the pressure of the hand or fingers to break down tension. The kneading, wringing, and friction strokes fall within this category.

Kneading: Kneading is both stimulating and relaxing, releasing tightness and tension, especially around the joints. It improves the circulation and lymph flow and helps to break down fatty tissue and aid the elimination of waste products from the body.

Action: With the fingers and thumbs of both hands, pick up muscle tissue away from the bone and compress tissue against tissue in an alternate, circular movement combined with a squeezing, slightly twisting action as you pass the gathered muscle tissue from hand to hand.

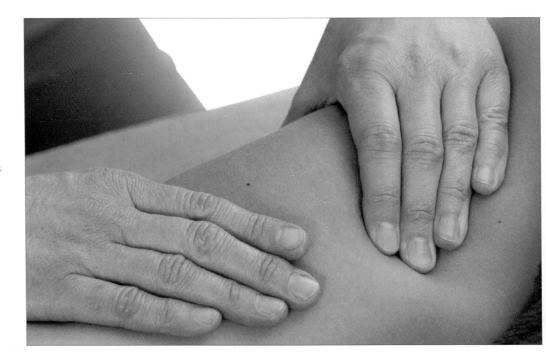

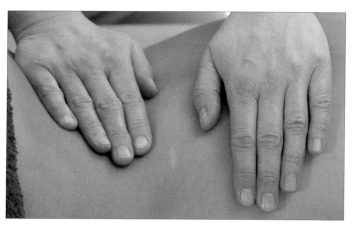

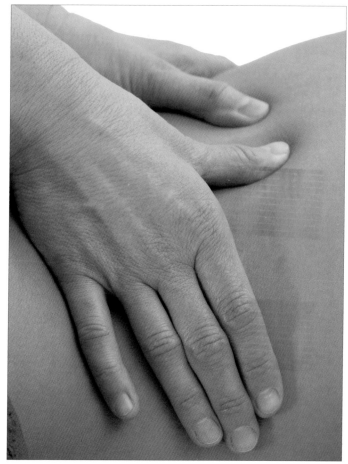

Wringing (above): The wringing stroke uses firm, rhythmic pressure. It is stimulating and relaxing, improves circulation and lymphatic drainage, and enlivens skin tissue. It is performed mostly on the back and the limbs.

Action: The action is literally one of "wringing" the muscle tissue. Start with both hands together and parallel. Slide your hands away from each other to each edge of the area you are massaging. Then slide them back to meet in the middle, where the tissue is twisted together in a stimulating (but not painful) way, before sliding apart again. Repeat in a vigorous, but smooth, continuous rhythm.

Friction (right): The name of this stroke derives from the Latin *fricare*, which means to rub. It is a deep, penetrative stroke used specifically on a small area. The friction action heats up the local area, improves circulation, promotes lymph drainage, stimulates the nerves, and releases tension by stretching muscle fibers.

Action: With the balls of the thumbs or pads of the fingers, apply firm pressure using your body weight. Circle the tissue immediately below the thumbs or fingers slowly and deeply, pressing the tissue over the bone rather than sliding your thumbs over the skin tissue.

percussion

Percussion derives from the Latin word *percutere*, which means to hit. The hacking and cupping strokes below are percussive strokes.

Hacking: Hacking uses the hands or fingers and is brisk, invigorating, and stimulating.

Action: The hacking action is achieved by using the edge of the hand or fingers in a fast, rhythmical chopping motion. Hands and fingers should be relaxed and strike the body (usually the more fleshy areas) with alternate strokes, originating from the wrists, with relaxed arms and shoulders. Begin with light, slow pressure and build up to a vigorous rhythm.

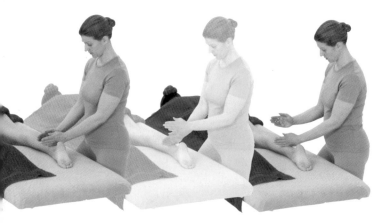

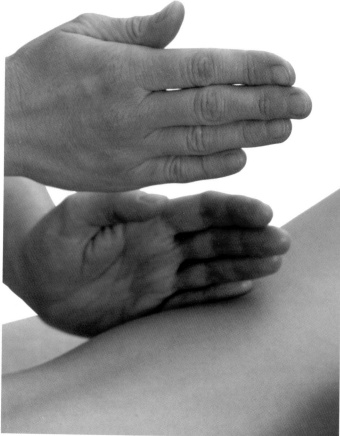

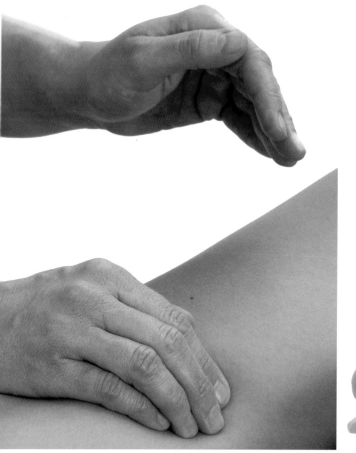

Cupping: In this stroke, the hands are cupped and fingers pressed together to create a suction vacuum. Cupping stimulates the nerve endings, warms the tissue, tones the muscles, and draws blood to the surface of the skin. It is a warming, invigorating, and stimulating action.

Action: Begin slowly with light pressure and build up to a vigorous rhythm with firm pressure and a feeling of creating suction against the skin. Keep both hands and wrists relaxed and the movement brisk and springy. Correct cupping produces a sound like a horse trotting.

starting the massage

Before you begin, find out how your partner is feeling and note any physical issues or problems. Before leaving the room to allow them to undress, give them the covering towel, ask them to lie on their front, indicate the direction in which you wish them to lie, and ask them to cover themselves ready for your return. Wash your hands before the massage.

With your partner still covered by the towel, face your partner's left side and start the massage with a hold, bringing your right hand to rest gently on the sacrum (the area in the center of the spine just above the buttocks) and your left hand to the center of the spine, at the top of the shoulders below the neck. If your partner is lying askew and not in balance, make adjustments to the body. These adjustments are important as they will align and balance the body and mind in preparation to receive the massage, an important step in bringing balance to the body and mind before the massage even begins. Carry out the front of the body adjustments (overleaf) when your partner has turned over.

Fold the towel down to expose the back down to buttock level and apply sufficient oil to your hands to cover the back area with a very thin film. Your hands should slide easily but not slither. Apply the oil to your partner's back with the effleurage stroke, and begin. Enjoy!

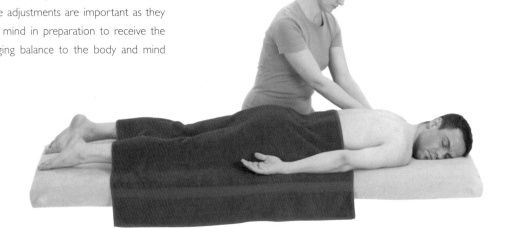

back of the body adjustments: arm stretch

Place both hands around the upper arm at shoulder level and, with a long, slow stretch, slide your hands down the arm with a sense of releasing the shoulder, elbow, and wrist joints. Take the stretch right out through the hand and fingers. Repeat on the other side.

shoulder stretch
With your left leg forward and right leg back, place your hands on the shoulders, stretching and releasing them by leaning your body weight through straight, strong arms.

Slowly release and finish this adjustment by sliding your hands around the shoulders, up the back of the neck, and out the head.

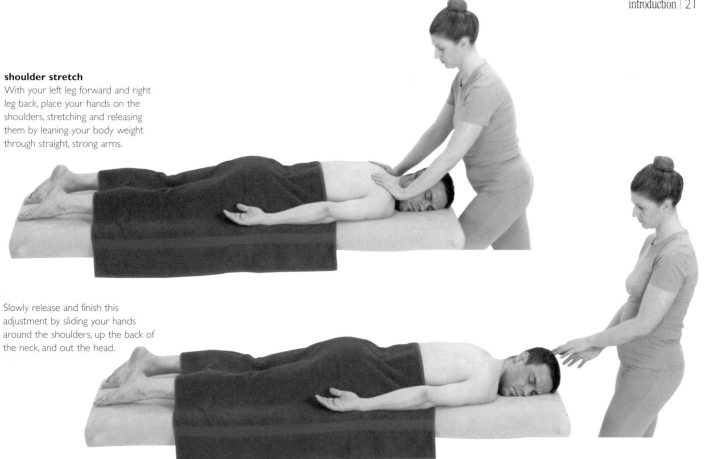

front of the body adjustment

Grasp the feet under the ankles and, with straight arms, lean back, giving the legs a long, slow, deep stretch as you do. Imagine the stretching releasing the joints all the way down the legs from hips to ankles. Slowly release and lower the feet on to the couch.

arm stretch

As in the back adjustment, start from the shoulder, using both hands, to create a long, slow stretch down the entire arm and out the hand and fingers.

neck stretch

Slide your hands under the base of the skull. Again, leaning back with straight arms and using your body weight, gently stretch the neck, bringing your hands out under the head.

go with the flow

The special Flowmotion images used in this book have been created to ensure that you can see each stage of every exercise and not just isolated highlights. Each sequence is shown across the page from left to right, demonstrating how the move progresses and develops safely and effectively, and is accompanied by clear, concise, step-by-step captions.

Below this, another layer of information in the timeline breaks the move into its various key stages, with various instructions indicating when to, for example, "use body weight," "flexible wrists," and "straight arms." The symbols in the timeline also include instructions for when to pause and when to move seamlessly from one stage to the next.

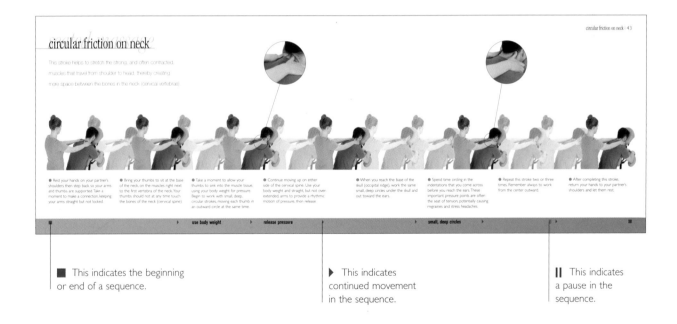

This indicates the beginning or end of a sequence.

This indicates continued movement in the sequence.

This indicates a pause in the sequence.

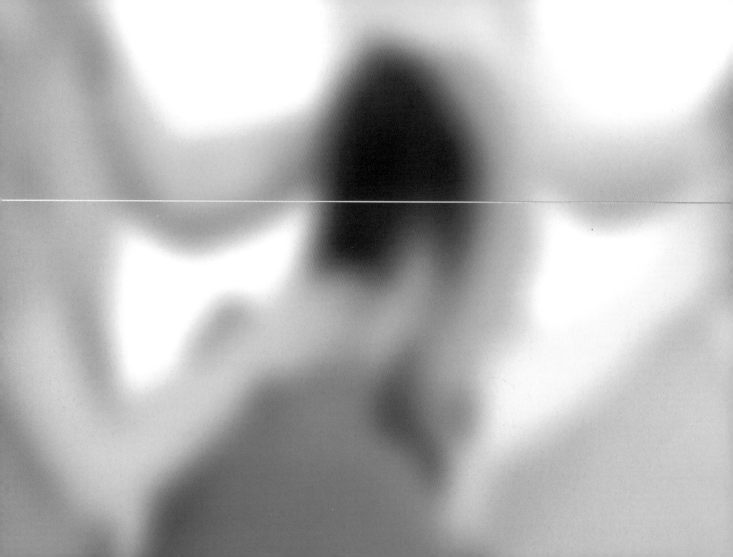

seated massage

kneading shoulders and back

Shoulders, in particular, and backs bear the brunt of the burdens of a modern stressful life and are often the source of irritability, tension, and migraine headaches. This simple kneading stroke can quickly and effectively release tension and induce a real feeling of relaxation.

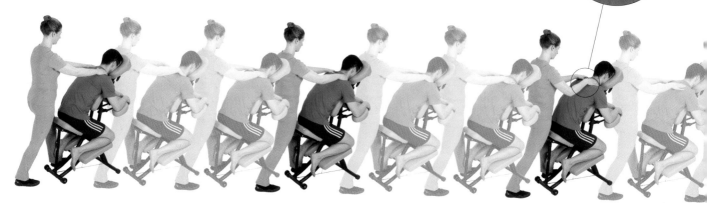

● Take a moment to center yourself and become aware of your breath. Step forward with your left foot and place your hands lightly on your partner's shoulders at the points where the neck and shoulders meet.

● Allow a few moments for your partner to get used to the feel of your hands and for a connection to be made between you.

● Grasp the top of the shoulders between your thumbs, fingers, and palms; then knead and roll the tissue between your thumbs and fingers.

● Continue squeezing the shoulders between your fingers and palms, at the same time working your thumbs with a circular motion between the spine and shoulder blades (scapulas).

use body weight ▶ ▶ **knead firmly** ▶

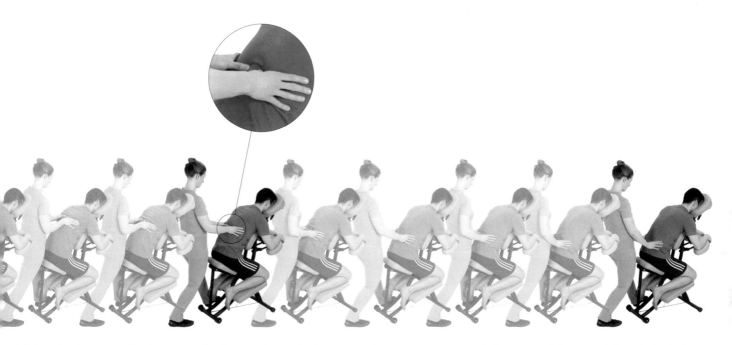

● Release the shoulders and, leaning with your body weight, make a circular motion with your thumbs, pressing into the muscle on either side of the spine (erector spinae).

● Continue working in a circular motion down beside the spine, moving about 1in (3cm) at a time. Use your body weight to sink your thumbs into the muscle tissue.

● Remember to lean your body forward when applying pressure, and to lean backward when you release the pressure.

● As you work down the back, adapt your posture by bending your knees. If you are comfortable, this will be conveyed to your partner. Complete this stroke as you reach the point just below the waist.

▶ **use deep pressure** ▶ ▶ ▶

circular effleurage beside spine

Although, technically, massage should not be used over the spine, this stroke is an exception in that its purpose is to provide a soft, soothing, and rhythmical rubbing to relax the nervous system.

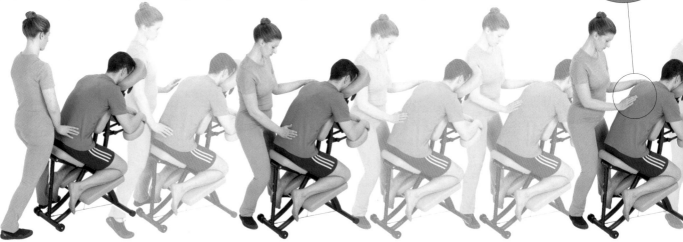

● After your hands come to rest on the lower back (sacrum) at the end of the previous stroke, move around to the left side of your partner.

● Bend your knees slightly for support and grounding; then place your left hand on your partner's left shoulder and your right hand in the middle of the lower back.

● Close your eyes for a moment to connect with your partner. This helps your partner to focus on the lower back area, a strong energy center (or chakra) of the body, and to prepare for the stroke.

● Keeping your right hand soft and flowing, begin to make gentle, encompassing circles in a clockwise direction over the spine.

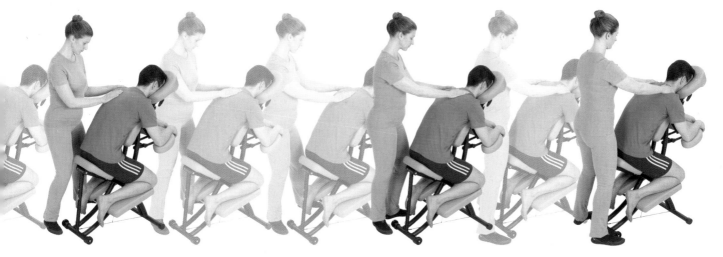

● It is most important that no pressure is exerted on the spine itself. Let your hand flow fluidly and gently over the contours of the area on which you are working.

● Continue this circular stroke, or effleurage, slowly working your way up your partner's spine. Make sure that you do not hurry this stroke. You can really take your time.

● Repeat this movement several times, working slowly and gently up and down the spine. Complete the sequence at the top of the back.

● Step back around to face your partner's back and bring both hands to rest on either side of the shoulders, near to the neck.

avoid spine   ▶   **use soothing strokes**   ▶   ▶   ▶

soft knuckle rubbing beside spine

This stroke is stimulating for both giver and receiver. It brings blood, energy, and nutrients to the surface of the skin, and warms and enlivens the tissue. It is performed with the loose, soft flat part of the knuckles.

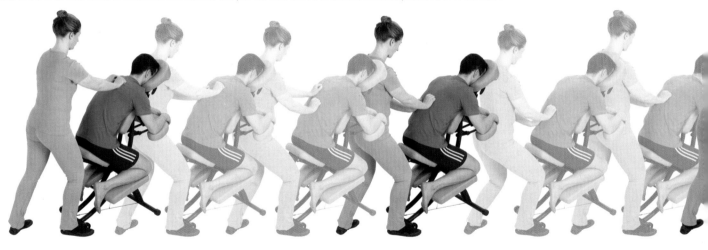

● Continuing from the last stroke, curl your hands into loose fists; then step back with one foot and place your hands at arm's length.

● Check that both of your knees are still bent slightly to give you support and grounding.

● Using a brisk, rubbing, up-and-down movement with alternate hands, begin at the top of the shoulders on the strong muscles (erector spinae) either side of the spine.

● Taking care not to touch the spine with the knuckles, continue working this brisk movement down toward the mid-back. Bend your knees to adjust your body height as you work.

▶   **soft, flat knuckles**   ▶   **brisk rubbing**   ▶   ▶

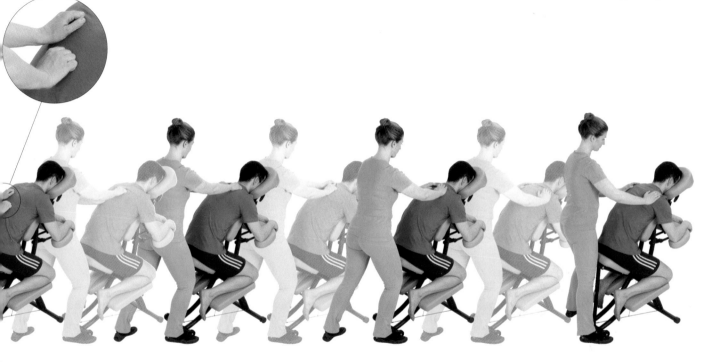

● Continue working the stroke with alternate hands until you reach just below your partner's waistline.

● Without stopping, reverse the procedure, using the same rubbing stroke to the mid-back.

● Continue up to the shoulders. You can repeat the movement two or three times.

● Bring your hands to the top of the shoulders. Finish off with soothing effleurage over the shoulders.

deep friction with forearm

The forearm is a useful and powerful tool in massage, particularly when used to stretch the strong muscle on top of the shoulder. Keep your wrist relaxed and your hand loose.

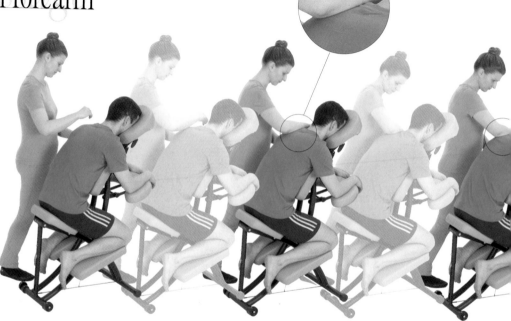

● Move to face the left side of your partner, positioning your body with the right leg back and left leg forward. Place your left hand on your partner's outer shoulder for support.

● Bend your right arm to 45 degrees, keeping your wrist and hand relaxed and loose. Place your mid-forearm where the neck meets the shoulder.

● Take a moment to make contact with your partner and allow your forearm to sink sensitively into the shoulder muscle.

● Using a deep, circular stroke in an outward direction, sink your body weight into the downward movement away from you and release the pressure as your forearm comes toward you.

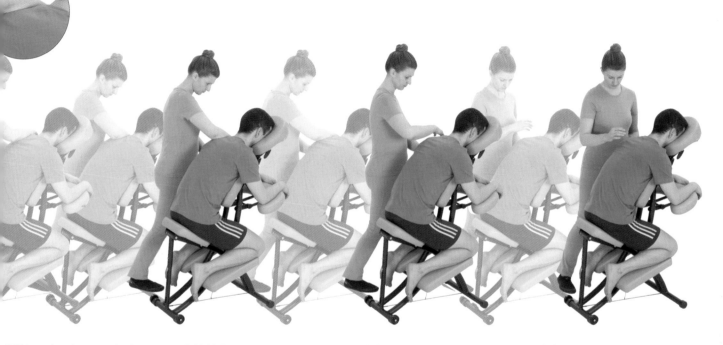

● This stroke releases tension in two powerful pressure points: one is sited on the shoulder, at two-fingers' width from the base of the neck, and the other sits just above the apex of each shoulder blade (scapula).

● Hold this position over the pressure points for the duration of five circles. Encourage feedback from your partner during the strokes.

● Continue with the same deep, circular movement, working slowly down the shoulder. Just before you touch the bony part of the shoulder, release your forearm.

● Step around to the left side of your partner, keeping your left hand supporting the shoulder.

heel of hand around shoulder blades

This stroke releases tension from the muscles in the upper back and neck.

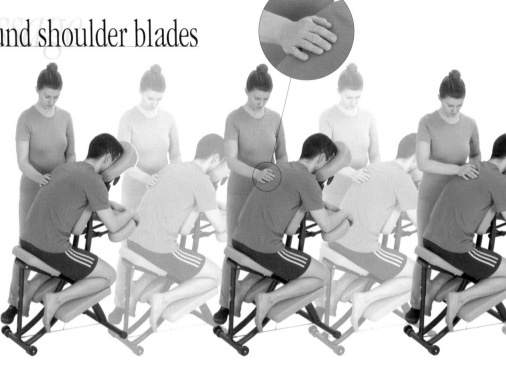

● With your left hand supporting your partner's left shoulder, place the heel of your right hand at the base of the left shoulder blade (scapula).

● Take your left foot back so that your body weight can flow to and fro to create pressure and release. Let the heel of your hand sink and stretch the muscle tissue, using the bony ridge of the shoulder blade as your guide.

● Allow time to sink deeply through superficial muscle (trapezius) into deeper muscle (rhomboid) before the stretch. As you work to mid-shoulder blade, imagine you are creating space between the shoulder blade and spine.

● Continue working slowly and steadily right around the shoulder blade, using the forward and backward, sinking and stretching motion. Work toward the top of the shoulder.

▶   **use body weight**   ▶   **stretch deep muscle**   ▶

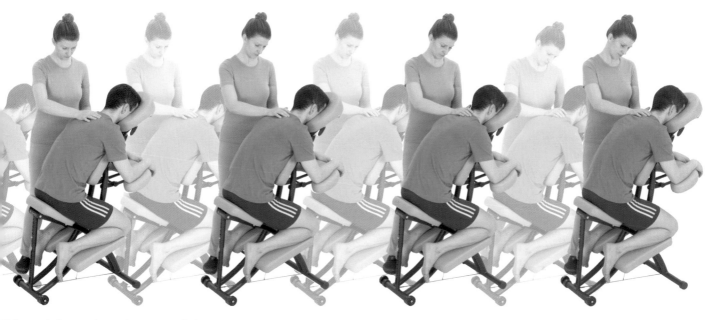

● Pay particular attention to the area at the top "corner" of the shoulder blade nearest the spine. This area is a major pressure point and is likely to be tense and sensitive, so encourage feedback from your partner.

● Continue the stroke around the top of the shoulder blade as far as you can go; then stop as soon as you touch bone.

● Rub the area you have just worked on with a gentle, soothing effleurage in a circular movement.

● Bring your right and left hands to either side of the shoulder to prepare you for the next stroke.

encourage feedback

squeeze down arm and hand

Our arms, which work for us ceaselessly—and thanklessly—respond gratefully to this simple stroke.

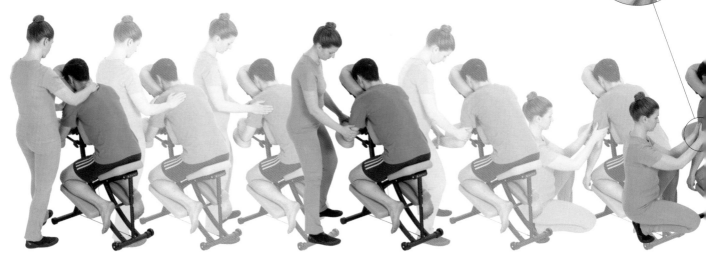

● Prepare for this stroke by placing your body into a comfortable position. Step your right leg back and place your hands either side of your partner's left shoulder.

● Supporting your partner's elbow with your right hand and the wrist with your left hand, gently lower the arm to hang down loosely at the side. Lower your body to accompany the arm by slightly bending your knees.

● Gently shake the arm to relax and prepare it for the stroke. Move into a kneeling position at this point.

● Grasp your partner's upper arm firmly between both hands, with your thumbs facing you. Squeeze down the arm with a flowing, rhythmic motion.

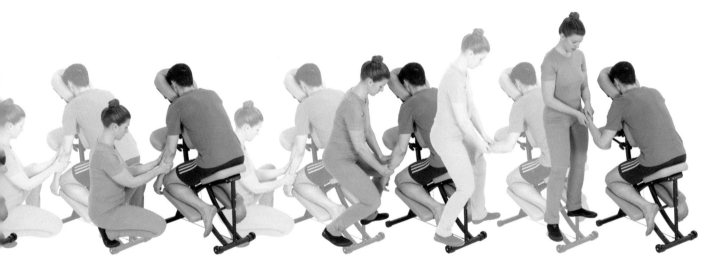

● Working down the upper arm, continue to squeeze and release it at about 1in (3cm) intervals.

● Move over the elbow and continue the stroke down the forearm, finishing at the hand. This stroke can be repeated until the tension is released.

● Take hold of your partner's hand with both hands and slowly lift the arm, rising to a standing position as you do so. Allow the arm to stay bent at the elbow.

● Clasp your hands loosely around your partner's hand; then use your thumbs and fingers to stretch, squeeze, and massage the hand fully.

knead and stretch hand and fingers

It is a luxury for our hard-working hands to be able to stop for a while and give themselves up to receiving, rather than doing and giving. This hand and finger massage will give them plenty of relaxing attention and will leave them feeling refreshed.

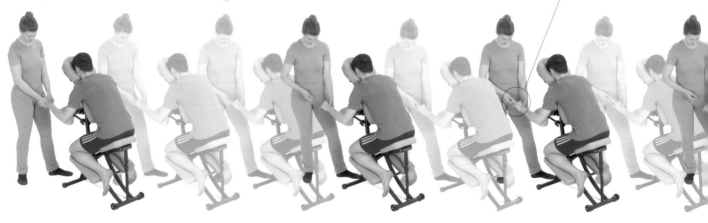

● Using your left hand to support your partner's right hand at the wrist, take the little finger between the thumb and fingers of your right hand.

● Begin to knead, squeeze, and roll the little finger before giving it a gentle pull and stretch; then release.

● Move on to the ring finger, giving it a good knead, roll, squeeze, and stretch. Keep the whole of your hand involved in the action. Remember to pay attention to the joints.

● Take the middle finger and, as before, encase it within your thumb, hand, and fingers to give it a good massage, roll, squeeze, and stretch.

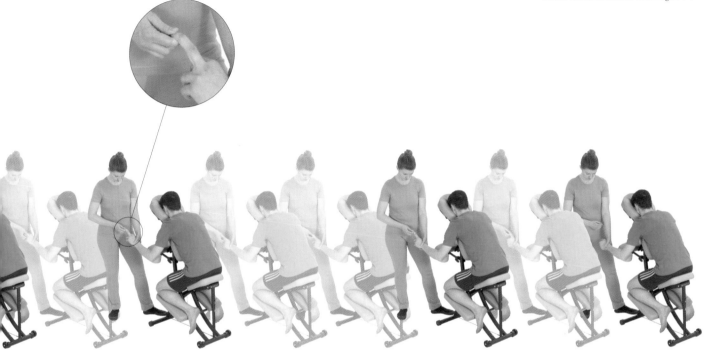

● Now massage the index finger. Roll and gently pull it; then stretch and release the finger.

● If you find it awkward to hold your partner's thumb, change your hands around and grasp the thumb with your left hand. Squeeze, roll, massage, and stretch the thumb; then release.

● Finish off the hand massage by kneading, squeezing, and stretching your partner's hand using both your hands.

● With your left hand still supporting your partner's left wrist, lower the arm in preparation for the next sequence.

knead thoroughly

brush off down arm

When muscle tissue is massaged or squeezed, the action releases energy. Brushing helps to disperse and clear this energy. This should be a light, feathering stroke.

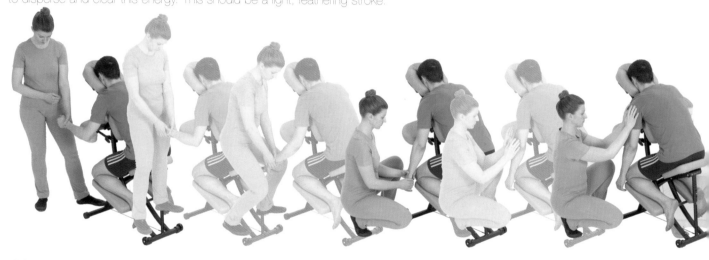

● Supporting your partner's hand with both hands, gently bring the arm to a relaxed position, allowing it to hang loosely at your partner's side.

● As you lower the arm, remember to adjust your position by bending your knees to lower your body.

● Come to a kneeling position and give your partner's arm a slight wiggle and shake to relax it further.

● Raise both your hands and place them lightly around the top of your partner's upper arm.

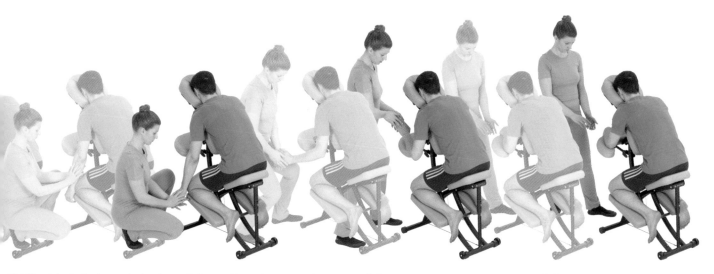

● With a light, feathering stroke, brush downward and outward along the entire arm and hand. As you work, imagine that you are dusting off and clearing released energy.

● Repeat this stroke three or four times, always working in a downward motion toward the hand.

● Enclose your partner's hand within your own hands and slowly rise to a standing position. Lift the hand as you rise and return it to its original position; then release.

● Step back and take a moment to reconnect with yourself. Repeat the whole of this sequence (starting on page 32) on your partner's right-hand side.

circular friction on neck

This stroke helps to stretch the strong, and often contracted, muscles that travel from shoulder to head, thereby creating more space between the bones in the neck (cervical vertebrae).

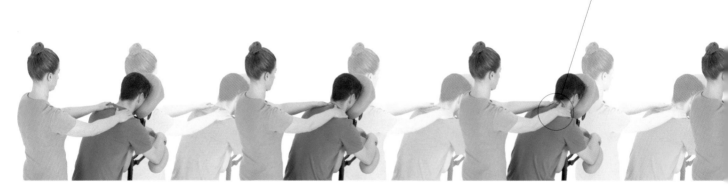

● Rest your hands on your partner's shoulders and then step back so your arms and thumbs are supported. Take a moment to make a connection, keeping your arms straight but not locked.

● Bring your thumbs to sit at the base of the neck, on the muscles right next to the first vertebra of the neck. Your thumbs should not at any time touch the bones of the neck (cervical spine).

● Take a moment to allow your thumbs to sink into the muscle tissue, using your body weight for pressure. Begin to work with small, deep, circular strokes, moving each thumb in an outward circle at the same time.

● Continue moving up on either side of the cervical spine. Use your body weight and straight, but not over-extended, arms to provide a rhythmic motion of pressure; then release.

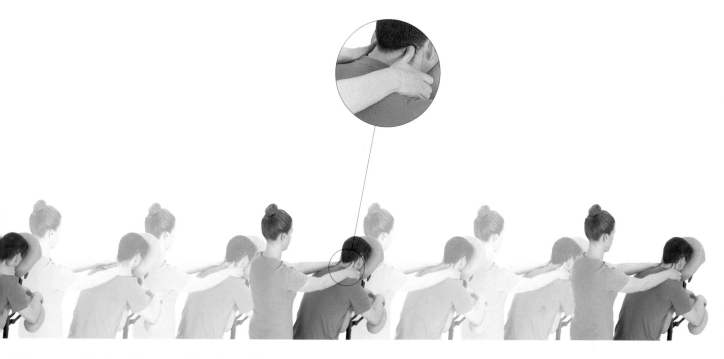

● When you reach the base of the skull (occipital ridge), work the same small, deep circles under the skull and out toward the ears.

● Spend time circling in the indentations that you come across before you reach the ears. These important pressure points are often the seat of tension, potentially causing migraines and stress headaches.

● Repeat this stroke two or three times. Remember always to work from the center outward.

● After completing this stroke, return your hands to your partner's shoulders and let them rest.

small, deep circles

circular friction on scalp

Scalp massage, as well as being very soothing, releases tension and encourages hair growth by relaxing the tiny muscles surrounding each follicle to create a freer flow of blood and nutrients to the area. After a stressful day at work, receiving a scalp massage can feel like heaven.

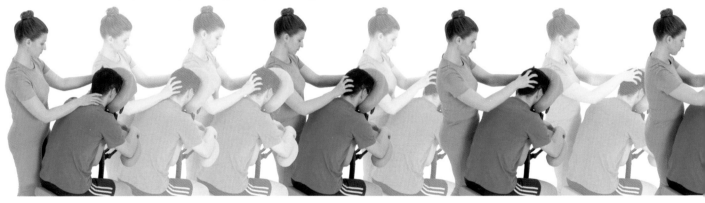

● Place your left hand just above your partner's eyebrows for support, and position your right hand at the base of the neck.

● Holding the fingers of your right hand quite rigidly, use the pads of your fingers to work small, deep circles in a clockwise direction, moving from the base of the skull up and around the back of the head.

● Rather than sliding your fingers over the surface of the head, use the pads of your fingers to grip the scalp firmly and slide them over the bones of the skull.

● Continue traveling over the sides and the top of the scalp, using the same circular movement. See if you can feel or sense any specific areas of tension.

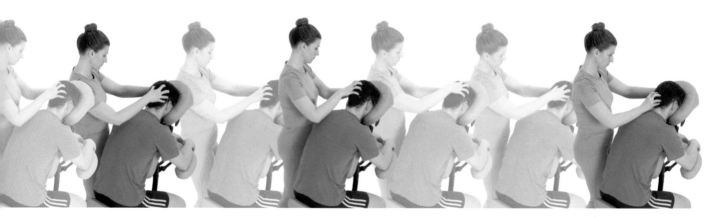

● Cover as much of the scalp as you can and encourage your partner to give you feedback as you work.

● Once you have covered the scalp with the deep friction stroke, try a lighter stroke by letting your finger pads travel over the surface of the scalp. This pleasing stroke stimulates the sebaceous glands that feed the hair follicles.

● Gradually bring the massage back to your starting point at the base of your partner's skull.

● Return your hands to your partner's shoulders and let them rest in preparation for the finishing sequence.

"washing hair" action

finishing sequence

This simple effleurage stroke, carried out slowly with intention, focus, and care, is a lovely way to complete a sequence. It helps to clear released energy and to soothe and balance the body and mind.

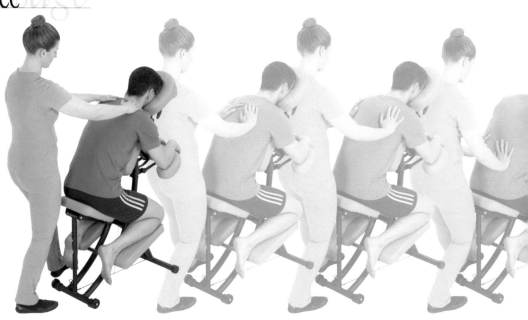

● Use a light stroke of the hands to "brush" off your partner's shoulders two or three times, clearing the body of released energy.

● Using the same "brushing" movement, gradually work across the top of the back.

● Continue this stroke, taking it down and across the back, then out to the sides of the body.

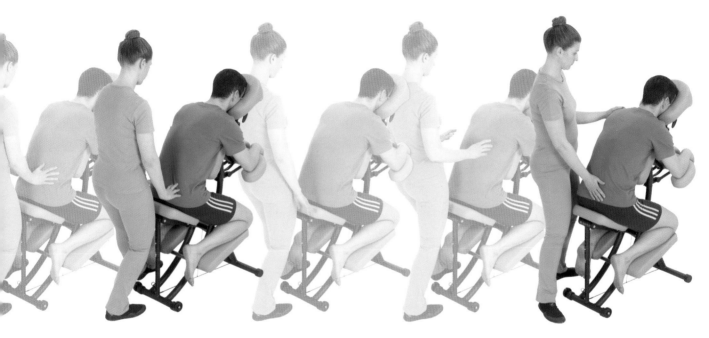

● Take care to brush your hands particularly softly over the kidney area, just above the waist.

● Work the brushing effleurage movement below the waistline, taking it to the lower back. Remember to bend your knees more, as you lower your body into a comfortable position.

● Return to a standing position to carry out a completion hold. Place your right hand on the lower back (sacrum) and your left hand on your partner's left shoulder.

● Close your eyes and imagine your two hands making a connection. When you feel your partner becoming still and peaceful, step back and take a few quiet, still moments to connect back to yourself.

take care over kidneys ▶ ▶ ▶ **stillness and focus** ■

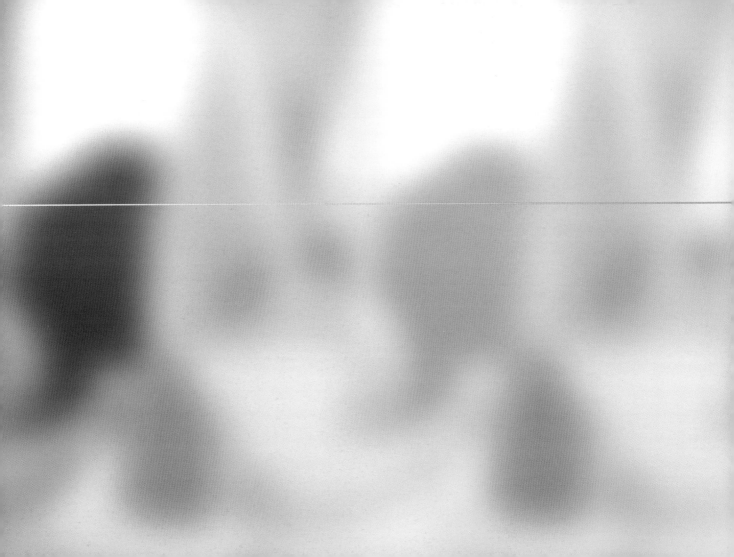

body massage

effleurage back and arms

The back is the largest expanse of body and the first area to be massaged. Remember that this will be your first contact with your partner and the first time that they experience your touch and its quality, so take time to center yourself, fold back the towel, oil your hands, and bring them slowly and softly on to the lower back (sacrum).

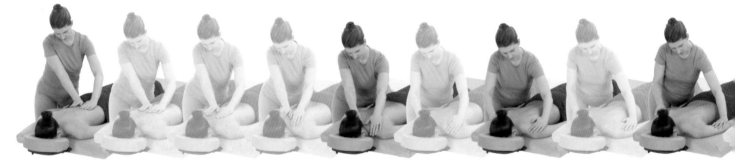

● The effleurage movement is used to oil the back and arms as well as provide the first massage stroke. Let the weight of your stroke be firm and smooth, and re-oil your hands whenever necessary.

● Keep your arms straight (but not locked), using your body weight to move them. Slide your hands, with even pressure, slowly up the back, on either side of the spine, to the shoulders.

● Continue sliding your hands over and around the shoulders. Aim to keep the movement fluid and smooth.

● Moving on from the shoulders, let your hands flow over and down the arms, encompassing the hands and fingers.

use body weight ▶ **even pressure** ▶

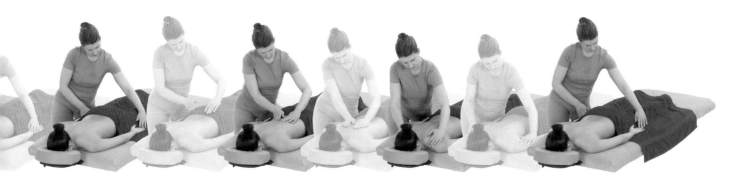

● Bring your hands back to their original position at the base of the spine. Oil your hands again, if necessary, and then repeat the stroke.

● The effleurage stroke can be carried out in the same area just beside the spine or taken outward at 1in (2.5cm) intervals in order to cover and oil the whole back.

● Gradually take the stroke up and around your partner's shoulders and out to the arms and hands.

● The whole stroke can be performed several times in order to cover the back well with oil. It also provides a calming and soothing beginning to the whole massage.

use flowing hands

sacrum stretch

The sacrum (also called the lower back) is the bony area directly above the buttocks which can often hold pain and tension. This stroke helps to stretch and lengthen the muscles covering the area, thereby making more space for the sacral and pelvic bones to settle more naturally. Do not use this stroke if the recipient has suffered a previous injury or bone degeneration.

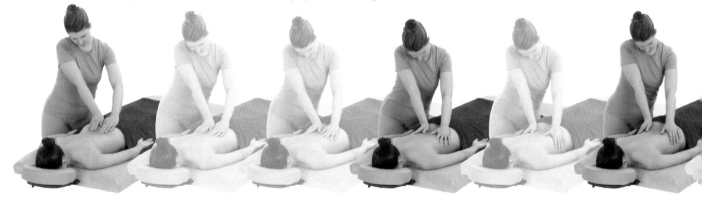

● Begin with your hands parallel and placed together at the top of the division of the buttocks. Lean your body weight forward through straight (but not locked) arms to the heels of your hands.

● As you slowly slide the heels of your hands apart, imagine that you are stretching the underlying muscle and widening the lower back.

● Although the pressure comes from the heels of the hands, the whole hand is engaged in the stroke, with your palms and fingers following the contours of your partner's body.

● Take the stroke as far as you can reach over the pelvis; then circle around the buttocks toward the hips, in a single motion in a downward circle.

■   **use body weight**   ▶   **straight arms**   ▶

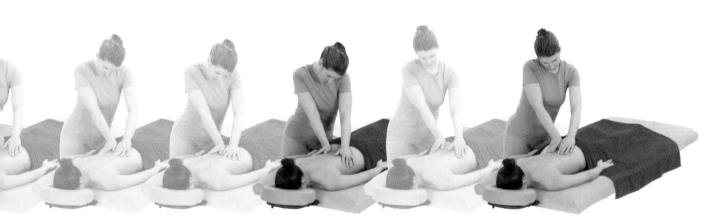

● Place your hands so that they are ½in (1cm) above their original position at the top of the buttock division. Begin another slow, deep stretch and circle.

● Slide the heels of your hands deeply through the muscles and continue working toward the hips in a circular movement. Encourage your partner to give you feedback so that you can apply the correct pressure.

● Repeat this stroke three times, starting each stroke ½in (1cm) above the previous position, to take your hands to the top of the pelvis.

● Bring your hands back to the original parallel position, ready to start the next part of the sequence.

▶ **heels of hands** ▶ ‖ ▶ ▶

wide circles from spine to sides

This is a lovely effleurage stroke because of its encompassing nature and the fact that it helps to include and integrate the sides of the body with the back. Move your body backward and forward to achieve depth, a good rhythm, and synchronize the movement with your breath.

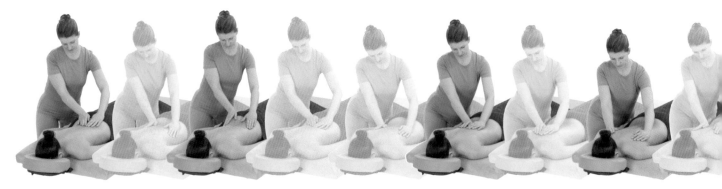

● Begin with the position of the previous stroke. Stand parallel to your partner, with your hands parallel beside the spine; then lean and sink your body weight into your hands.

● Keeping your arms straight but not locked, begin to slide your hands up the back. Make sure that your elbows are not allowed to collapse.

● After a short upward movement, make a wide, generous circle with your hands, covering the back and the sides of your partner's body.

● Bring your hands back to the original position just beside the spine, still keeping the movement going.

straight arms ▶ **wide circle** ▶ **use body weight** ▶

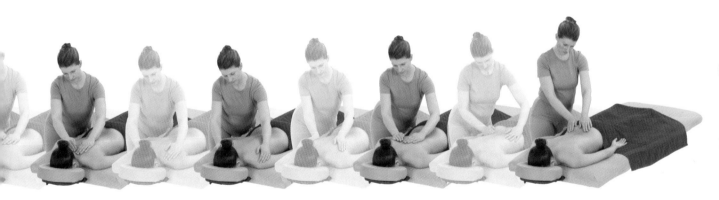

● Slide your hands to about 2in (5cm) above the original starting point.

● Keep the momentum of the circular movement smooth and continuous as you travel up the back and the sides of the body. Focus on working in deep, rhythmic circles.

● When you reach the shoulders, repeat the same stroke in a downward direction until you reach the original starting point.

● Keeping your hands in contact with your partner, turn your body to face across your partner in preparation for kneading on the left side.

continuous movement

kneading left side

The kneading stroke, akin to kneading bread, is deep and powerful. It has the advantage of being both stimulating (bringing energy and blood to the area) and relaxing because of its decongestant and tension-releasing action, bringing suppleness and pliability to the muscles. Firmly pick up as much tissue as you can and reach as much depth and penetration as your hands can manage.

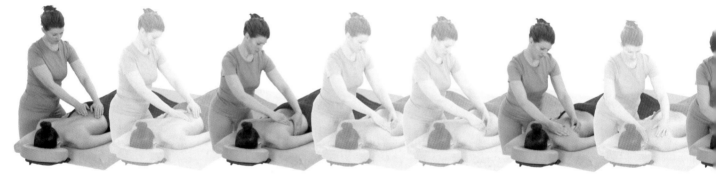

● Position your body to face your partner, keeping your knees bent and arms straight without locking them. You should be reaching with your arms across the body but not bending from the waist.

● Begin the kneading stroke on the fleshy part of the left buttock (the gluteals). Work on the strong muscles of the buttocks and build up a good dancing rhythm, using your whole body as well as your arms and hands.

● Keep the rhythm going as you work up from the buttock and along the side of your partner's body.

● Continue to knead up the side of the body and on top of the shoulder, seeking out and massaging as much tissue as possible, as you reach the ribcage and shoulder blades.

▶   **vigorous action**   ▶   **rhythm**   ▶   **depth**   ▶

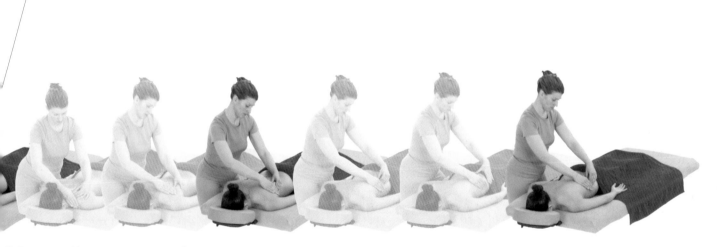

● Carry on working up the body until you reach the outside of the shoulder blades and the crease of the arm. Knead this area thoroughly, including the top of the shoulder.

● Without stopping the kneading movement, begin the return journey down the body to the starting point.

● Once you have reached the buttocks, spend some additional time working on this area.

● Bring your hands back to the parallel position where, ideally, you will continue seamlessly into the cupping stroke.

cupping stroke left side

Cupping is derived from an ancient technique for bringing blood to the surface of the skin. It warms the skin, tones the muscles, improves local circulation, is stimulating, and is pleasant to receive.

● Shape your hands into a cup, keeping your fingers firmly together. Place your cupped hands ½in (1cm) apart from each other and 1in (2.5cm) above the left buttock.

● Begin the brisk, percussive movement, which should have the "clopping" sound of a trotting horse. Start slowly and build up to a very fast rhythm. Practice will help you to perfect this technique.

● After spending some time on the buttock, begin working up the left side of your partner's back.

● Lighten the stroke as you reach and pass over the kidneys (the area between the top of the hips and the beginning of the ribcage).

▶   **start slowly**   ▶   ▶ **lighten the stroke**   ▶

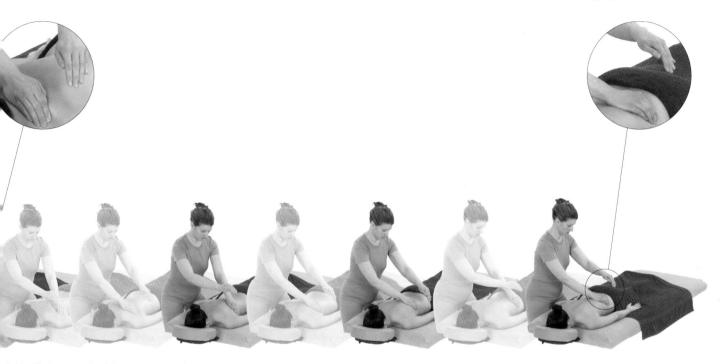

● Modify the strength of the stroke as you pass over the ribs and the shoulder blades. Increase the strength of the stroke as you reach the top of the shoulder.

● Continue all the way up to the shoulder. Pay special attention when cupping over the area between the shoulder and the neck (trapezius), which can often be contracted and very tense.

● Keep the rhythm going as you begin to make the return journey, working down the side to the buttock.

● When you reach the buttock you can continue straight into the hacking stroke, over the page.

hacking stroke left side

The hacking stroke, despite its fearsome name, is an effective and surprisingly pleasant stroke to receive. The benefit of this stroke is that it can reach and relax, on a vibrational level, muscle tissue that may be too dense and contracted to be penetrated using other strokes. The secret of effective hacking is a sharp, brisk, percussive, and vibratory action.

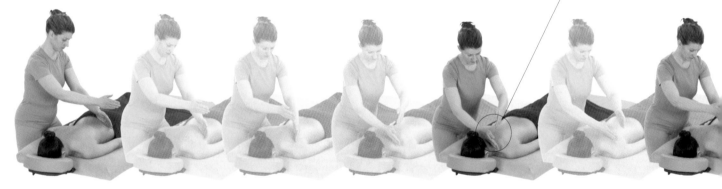

● From the previous position, bring the palms of your hands parallel to each other about 1in (2.5cm) and 2in (5cm) above your partner's body.

● Begin the hacking stroke on the left buttock, visualizing the action sending vibrations deep into the muscle tissue. Spend time on this area.

● Continue the hacking motion up the side of the body, keeping the pressure very light as you pass over the kidneys (between the top of the hips and the start of the ribcage).

● The hacking stroke is generally more effective over muscle tissue, so modify the pressure as you pass over the ribcage and shoulder blades. Increase the pressure as you reach the top of the shoulder.

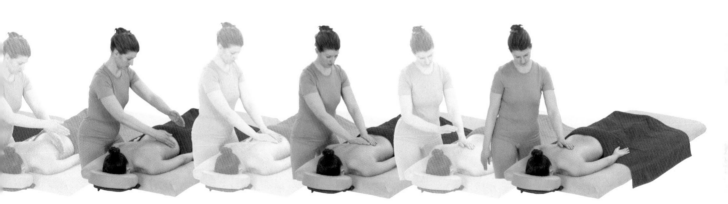

● Once you reach the shoulder, continue hacking over the shoulder muscle. Without stopping the motion, begin the return journey down the side of the back.

● Take care as you pass over the bony structures and the kidney area. When you reach the left buttock, spend time again on this dense muscle tissue.

● To compensate for and to provide a contrast to the stimulation and vigor of this stroke, place both hands on the middle of your partner's back, close your eyes, and allow a stillness to settle and manifest.

● Keeping one hand in contact with your partner, move to the other side and repeat the kneading, cupping, and hacking sequences on the right side. Return to the left side to start the thumb friction up and down the spine.

▶ **take care over kidneys** ▶ **stillness** ▶ ■

thumb friction up and down spine

Thumb friction, a deep and penetrative, small circular stroke, is performed to relax and decongest the long muscles beside the spine, which often become tight and tense in the struggle to survive and succeed. With this sequence, make sure that your thumbs do not touch the spine itself.

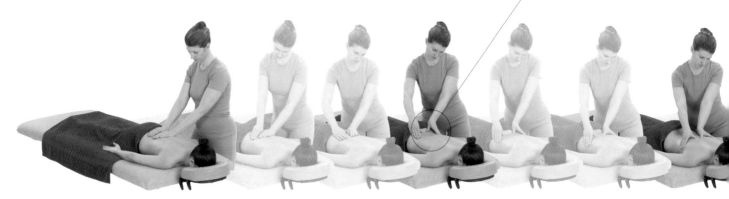

● Let your hands come to rest on the lower back. Facing your partner's left-hand side, turn your body to look up the back.

● Position your hands with your thumbs on either side of your partner's spine, just above the line of the pelvis. Check that your arms are straight but not locked, and have your left foot forward and right foot back.

● Lean your body weight forward and exert pressure through your thumbs, allowing them to sink into the muscle tissue. Move them in a small circle; then lean back, withdrawing your pressure and body weight.

● In a continuous motion of leaning forward into the circle and backward to release pressure, begin to work up the sides of the spine at 1in (2.5cm) intervals. Use lighter pressure in the space between the pelvis and ribs.

use body weight ▶ pressure and release ▶

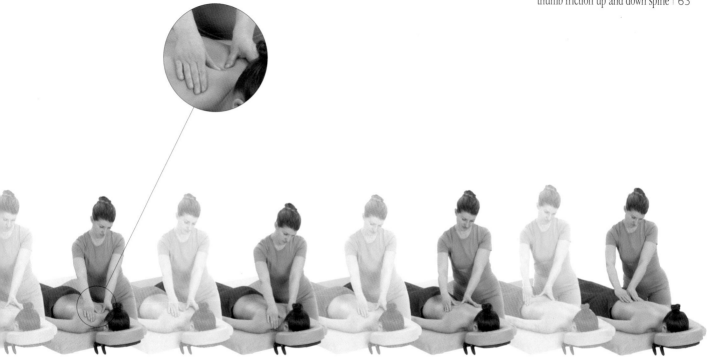

● Once you pass the unsupported area between the pelvis and ribs, the pressure can become deeper. Take your time and let your body enjoy the rhythm of this stroke.

● Continue to work the stroke all the way up to the top of your partner's back. Then, without stopping, begin the return journey to your starting point.

● Remember to use your body weight to maintain deep pressure with your thumbs. Again, use lighter pressure on the area between the pelvis and ribs.

● Bring your hands to a parallel position on either side of the spine, ready to effleurage to the "kneading shoulder" stroke.

kneading the shoulders

Because the shoulders often become a repository for stress and tension, the kneading stroke alleviates any discomfort as it works deeply into two sets of pressure points.

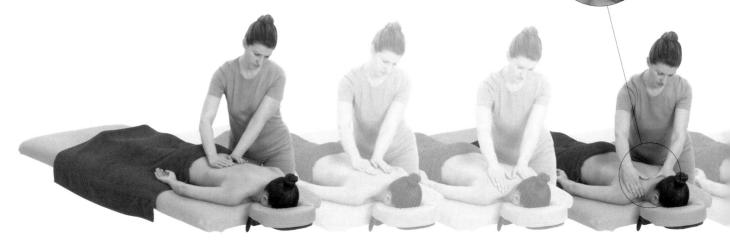

● Continue from the last stroke, starting at the base of the spine, and effleurage to the mid-back. Keep your hands and fingers relaxed and, at the same time, in firm contact with your partner's body.

● Continue to effleurage up to your partner's shoulders, keeping your arms straight and strong, but not locked. Shift your body weight and, if necessary, your feet to avoid leaning forward awkwardly.

● On reaching the shoulders, grasp the shoulder muscle deeply between fingers, thumbs, and the palms of your hands, picking up the tissue away from the underlying bone and squeezing it between fingers and thumbs.

● When working this deep stroke, check with your partner as tolerance to pressure can vary. Knead both shoulders simultaneously with left and right hands working in the same forward and backward rhythm.

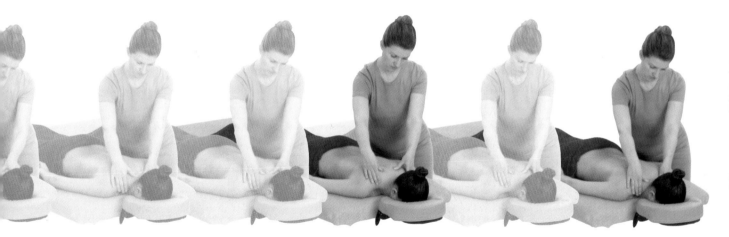

● Make sure you are familiar with the pressure points. The first is located two-fingers' width from the neck on top of the shoulders; the second is at the top "corner" of the shoulder blade nearest to the neck.

● If preferred, you can alternate the stroke by using the left hand to pick up the tissue as the right hand gradually releases it, and vice versa.

● Remember to take care of your wrists and thumbs while you are massaging. Always stop or modify the massage if they become tired, painful, or start to feel overused.

● Bring your hands to rest at the top of your partner's shoulders before proceeding to the next stroke.

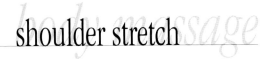
shoulder stretch

This stroke is a variation on the shoulder kneading stroke shown on pages 64–65. As the name suggests, it gives the shoulders and trapezius muscle a very effective, releasing stretch.

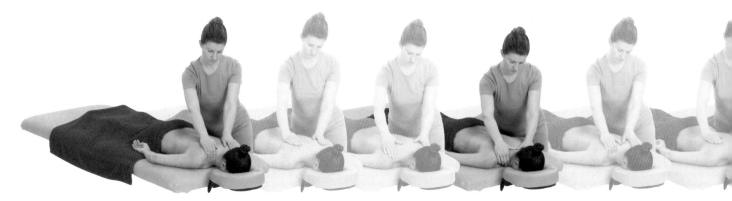

● For the shoulder stretch you will need to assume a solid stance. Stand with your left leg forward and your right leg back, and use straight, strong arms as you perform this stroke.

● Using the whole of your hands, fingers, and thumbs, take hold of your partner's shoulders. Ask your partner to relax and to take a deep breath in and out. Synchronize your breathing with that of your partner.

● When both of you are breathing out, shift your weight from the front to the back leg, pulling back with your hands to stretch the shoulder muscle. On the out breath, lean forward to prepare for the next stretch.

● Repeat the shoulder stretch several times. Encourage your partner to resist the urge to "help" you by lifting the shoulders, as your partner's body weight is necessary to make this an efficient stretch.

▶ **strong stance** ▶ **inhale then exhale** ▶ ▶

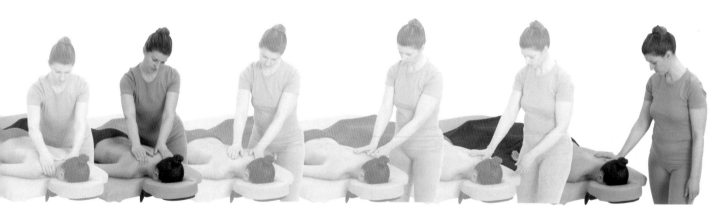

● Relax your hands and release your partner's shoulders. Now give a soothing effleurage over the area that you have just worked on.

● Still working with gentle effleurage, gradually move your hands over the top of your partner's back.

● Adjust your position so that you are facing across your partner's back, with your hands resting lightly over the upper back. Then release your left hand and move around the top of your partner's head.

● Place your left hand on the right shoulder and your right hand on the left shoulder. Take a few deep breaths, and then slowly lift your hands away. Move down to the sacrum to start the wringing stroke.

effleurage

wringing stroke

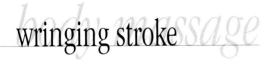

The wringing stroke, although stimulating to the skin, has a very soothing and relaxing effect on the body and mind, with its gentle rhythmic, rocking, and encompassing action.

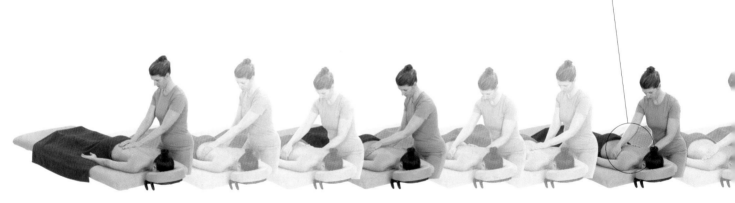

● Bring your hands to rest together on the sacrum, the starting position for the wringing stroke.

● Pull your right hand and arm toward you at the same time as you push your left hand and arm away from you. Notice a feeling of grip and twist to the skin as you alternate the pulling of your hands.

● Take your time with this stroke, traveling slowly up the back. Make sure that you keep your own body in an upright, relaxed position.

● As you "wring" and pull the back, include the sides, reaching as far as you can in order to integrate the often-forgotten sides of the body.

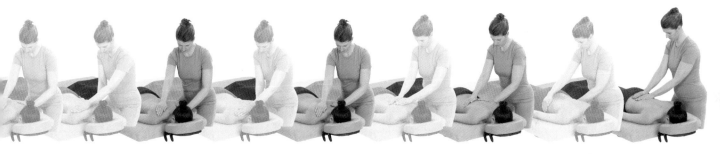

● Work all the way up to the crease of the arm, and then continue right up to your partner's shoulders.

● Without stopping the rhythm of the wringing stroke, begin the return journey to the sacrum. Finish the back massage with the same effleurage stroke with which you began.

● When you reach the lower back, rest your hands for a moment in the starting position to bring the back massage to a close. Cover your partner with a towel and prepare to work on the next area, the legs.

● To connect the back with the legs, go to the feet and place your hands on the soles, holding them there for a few moments. This is a powerful hold as the soles of the feet and the palms of the hands contain energy centers.

effleurage back of leg

This long, sweeping effleurage stroke is a lovely variation of the same action that opened the back massage but which is now adapted to the narrower expanse of the back of the leg. This action will relax and prepare the limb to receive the deeper strokes shown on the next pages.

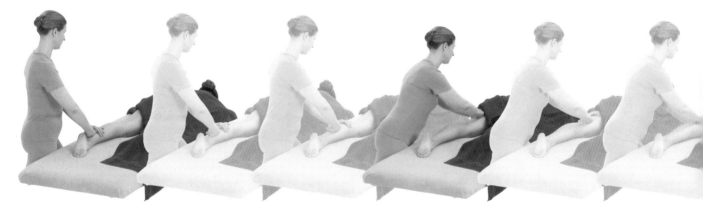

● Move down from the back, parallel with your partner's left side, and level with the foot. Fold back the towel to expose the whole of the left leg and oil your hands. Stand with your left leg forward and your right leg back.

● Keep your arms slightly rounded, but not collapsed, at the elbows. Place your right hand across the leg above the heel with the fingers pointing left. Place the left hand above with the fingers pointing right.

● Lean your body weight into your hands. Using your fingers and the whole of your hands, encompass the contours of your partner's leg and begin the slow, firm slide of the effleurage stroke.

● As your hands reach the top of the leg, circle your left hand outward around the hip bone. Rotate the right hand toward the inner thigh.

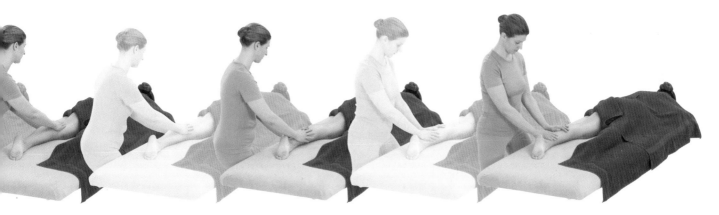

● Take the pressure off for the downward effleurage but use this opportunity to include a light stretch of the leg. Remember to re-oil your hands whenever the area you are massaging feels too dry.

● As you slowly pull and stretch the leg, allow your hands to follow the contours of the whole of the leg. During the effleurage stroke, make sure that you make full contact by using your whole hand.

● Continue working on the stretch down the left leg until you reach the area above the heel.

● Turn to face across your partner's leg and lightly rest your hands in front of you. Take a moment to prepare for the next movement.

foot massage

It is easy to forget about our feet and the great job they do daily. As the sole of the foot, according to reflexology, contains reflexes that connect and relate to the whole of the body, a foot massage can be beneficial and relaxing for the whole body and mind.

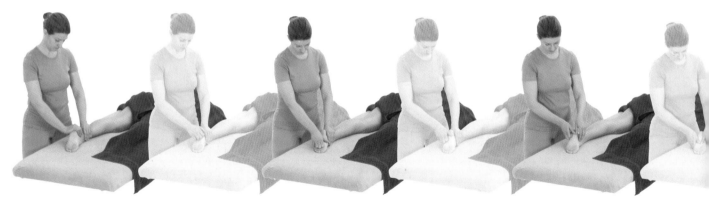

● Lightly oil your partner's foot. Turning to look down toward the toes, rest your left hand on the heel, and with your right hand, do a soft-knuckle stretch on the heel.

● Using your knuckles, make small, circular strokes over the heel and the sole of the foot, working as deeply as is comfortable for your partner. In reflexology, this area of the foot relates to the lower back.

● As you work downward over the heel and toward the sole of the foot, begin to use your fingers also to create a stretch and squeeze of the whole foot.

● Let your thumbs continue with the circular stroke, as you work firmly down the middle of the sole.

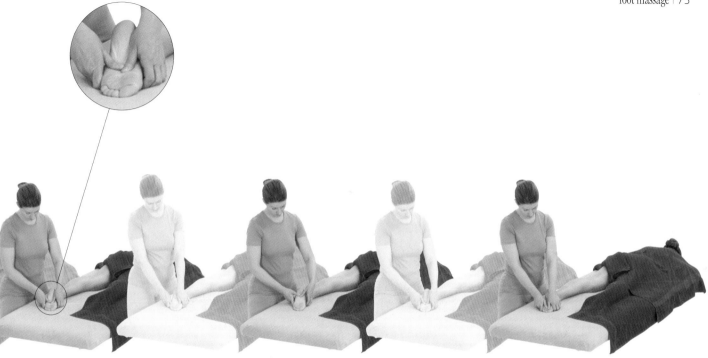

● Take the circular movement into the inner foot, working along the ridge of the instep, which, in reflexology, relates to the spine.

● Now take the massage to the outer ridge of the sole. Remember to keep the circular strokes firm.

● Work your thumbs in a circular movement around the pad of the sole (the area under the toes).

● Give the toes a squeeze with both hands before releasing your partner's foot, ready for the next stroke.

use circling thumbs ▶   ▶   ▶   ❚❚ ▶

toe massage

This massage, which completes the massage on the sole of the foot, gives breathing space to your toes.

In reflexology, the toes, and particularly the big toe, relate to all areas of the head, neck, and face.

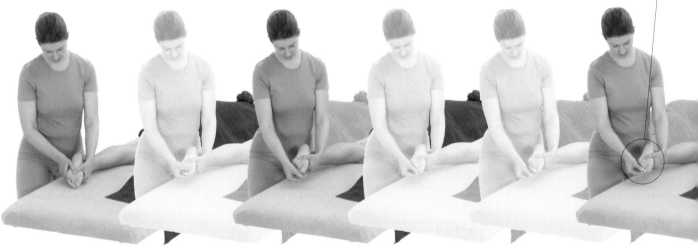

● Remaining in the same position as the previous page, support your partner's foot with your left hand and work with the thumb of your right hand underneath each toe.

● Start with the big toe on the left foot. Working in small circles, massage and stretch under the "neck" of the toe. Move on to the ball of the toe, with the same thorough treatment, and massage right out to the end of the toe.

● Move on to the middle toe, working with your thumb and fingers to massage and stretch it, and pulling out from the end of the toe to finish.

● Now take hold of the third toe and repeat the circular movement, working from the base of the toe to the top.

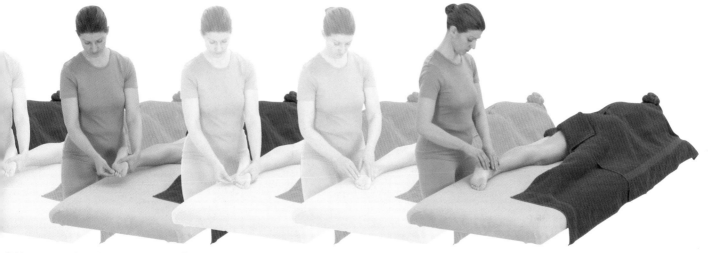

● Massage, stretch, and gently pull the fourth toe. As our feet are confined within shoes and socks most of the day, they can become energetically restricted. This massage will help to release that feeling of constriction.

● Finally, take hold of the little toe and massage with a circular movement; then pull and stretch the toe to finish.

● Grasping all five toes at the same time, give them a final squeeze.

● Turn to face across your partner's body and take a moment to prepare for the next stroke.

kneading back of leg

This stroke kneads the whole of the back of the leg, working into the strong muscles of the calf (gastrocnemius) and hamstrings, which are responsible for walking, running, sitting, and rising. They can often be tense and contracted but respond well to the deep action of the kneading stroke.

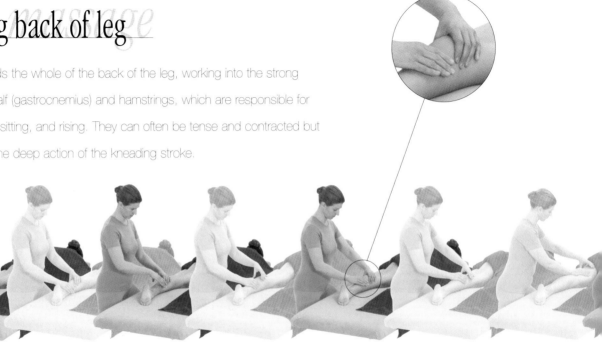

● Facing across your partner's left leg, lift both hands to lightly hold the lower leg, just above the heel, between your fingers and thumbs. Space your thumbs about 1in (2.5cm) apart.

● Start the kneading stroke by picking up muscle tissue between the fingers and thumb of your right hand and pushing it toward your left hand. Pick up the tissue with your left hand and feed it back to your right hand.

● Thoroughly knead the calf muscle in this way, using a rhythmic, continuous action. Allow your body to almost "dance" as you move your hands vigorously from side to side.

● As you work along the calf muscle, take care not to knead the area over the back of the knee.

▶ **knead from hand to hand** ▶ **rhythm and vigor** ▶ **work deeply** ▶

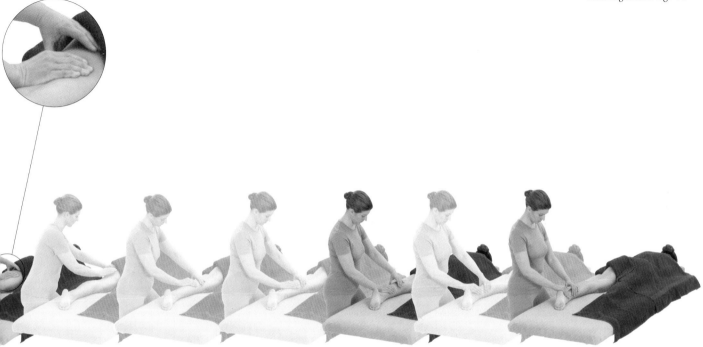

● When you reach the back of the thigh (the hamstrings), knead the inner, middle, and outer areas thoroughly.

● Continue to knead with a rhythmic action, working right up to the outer base of the buttocks.

● Without stopping, begin the return journey down the thigh and toward the lower leg. Remember to avoid kneading across the back of the knee.

● Let your hands come to rest briefly on your partner's lower leg above the heel before starting the next stroke.

▶ **"dance" your body** ▶ **avoid knee** ▶ ❚❚ ▶

cupping back of leg

This stimulating percussive stroke brings blood to the surface of the skin to revitalize the area

on which you are working, particularly where muscle tissue might be dense, cold, and contracted.

Cupping leaves the back of the leg feeling invigorated, alive, and pleasantly tingling.

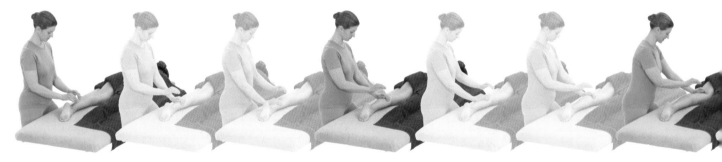

● Stand facing across your partner's left leg and position your hands together just above the heel.

● Form a cup with each hand, pressing your fingers together, and slowly begin the cupping action. Make sure that your hands stay close together and near to the leg.

● Your hands need to make a strong "clopping" (but never a slapping) sound, a little like a horse trotting. If your hands are correctly cupped, your partner will experience a strong but never painful sensation.

● Travel up the leg, letting the rhythm become faster and more staccato. This stroke should be as energizing and stimulating to you as it is to your partner. Ease off the pressure as you cup behind the knee.

▶ **form a firm cup** ▶ **start slowly** ▶ **brisk, even rhythm** ▶

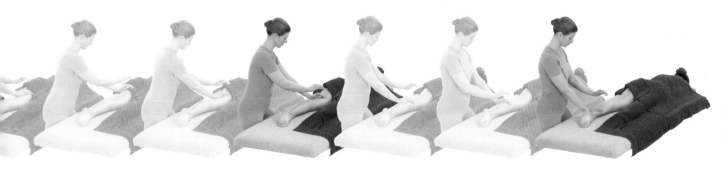

● Give each area you are cupping sufficient attention so that the tissue can become warmed and stimulated.

● On reaching the top of the thigh you can also continue over the covered buttock if you wish.

● Without stopping, and using the same brisk, cupping action, work your way down the leg, again easing the pressure over the back of the knee.

● Bring your hands back briefly to their original resting position before beginning the next stroke.

hacking back of leg

Sometimes the kneading stroke may not reach strongly enough into the "hamstrings" on the back of the thigh or the calf muscles if they are contracted and tense. In these cases, the hacking stroke is ideal as it uses vibration to stretch and relax the muscle fibers. Think of this stroke as having a "tenderizing" effect on the muscles.

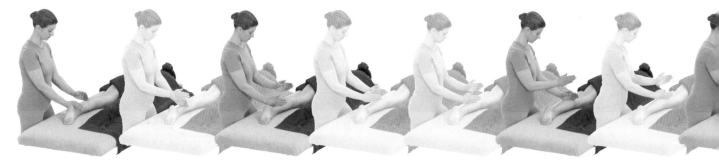

● Stand facing across your partner's left leg. Check that your knees are flexible rather than locked.

● Keeping the palms of your hands parallel and about ½in (1cm) apart, begin the stroke on the back of the calf just above the heel.

● With wrists flexible and making contact with the little fingers (you can use the edges of your hands on the hamstrings), start the hacking stroke. Work slowly to begin with.

● As you reach the calf muscle (gastrocnemius), make the stroke more rapid and brisk. Spend some time in this area as it can be tense. Ask your partner for feedback to assess how much pressure to apply.

▶ **start slowly** ▶ **flexible wrists** ▶ ▶

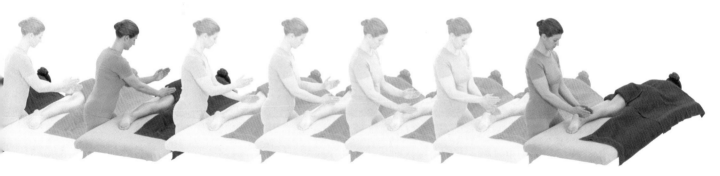

● Remember to avoid working across the back of the knee and simply move your hands across to the next area. Spend some time on the tough "hamstring" muscles, where you can use the edge of the hand.

● Remember to take into account the variation in muscle density from person to person. An athlete would need more attention to this area than, say, an office worker.

● Continue to hack over the covered buttock (the gluteals), another large area of strong muscle that benefits from this stroke. Then bring the stroke back down over the hamstrings, taking care to avoid the back of the knee.

● Work your way over the calf muscle and, finally, let your hands come to rest above the ankle. You are now ready to start the wringing stroke.

brisk and vigorous ▶ **use bouncing rhythm** ▶ ▶ ■

wringing back of leg

As the wringing stroke is most effective on the fleshier and more muscular parts of the body, the back of the leg responds well to this vigorous, but also soothing, stroke. Really get your body moving in a dancing rhythm as your hands slide backward and forward, meeting in the middle with a good stimulating twist to the skin.

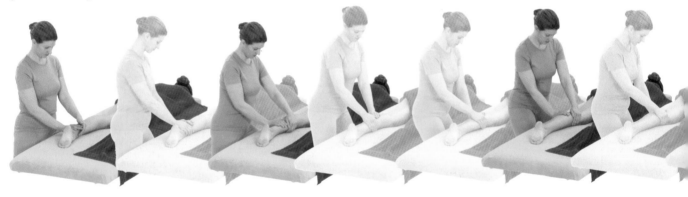

● Stand facing across your partner's left leg with your knees flexible. Your hands will already be in position to begin the wringing stroke on your partner's left ankle.

● As one hand moves away from you, the other moves toward you, as if you were "wringing" a towel. Aim to get a good painless skin stretch going as your hands meet back in the middle.

● Keeping your knees flexible, move your body rhythmically with this energetic stroke.

● Wringing is an encompassing, generous stroke, so slide each hand to each side of the leg as far as it will go. When your hands return to meet in the middle, try lifting the muscle tissue to get a good stretch and twist.

flexible knees ▶ **stretch and twist**

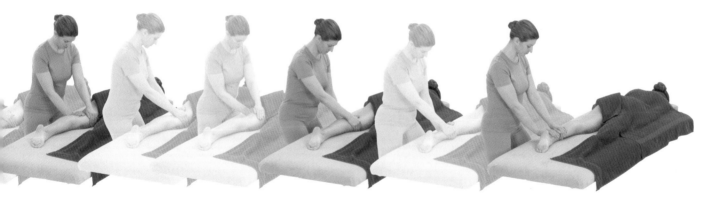

● Work lightly over the back of the knee; then resume a stronger pressure as you reach the "hamstrings" on the back of the thigh.

● Continue to wring with a rhythmic movement, until you reach a suitable stopping point on the inner thigh. Stay in that area while you complete the stroke up the outer thigh, with the left hand.

● Without stopping, begin the downward journey, using the same rhythm and pressure. Again, remember to release the pressure as you work across the back of the knee.

● Continue to wring over the calf muscle and down to the ankle. Bring your hands to rest just above the heel.

use dancing rhythm

effleurage stroke on back of leg

Because effleurage is a soothing, relaxing, and encompassing stroke, it can also be used at the end of a sequence to integrate the massage and to relax the recipient after a series of deeper and more vigorous strokes has been applied.

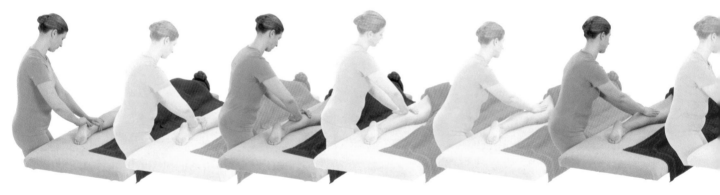

● Stand on your partner's left side, facing toward the head. Place your hands across each other. In this stroke, the upper hand is always the outside hand (whichever leg). This lets your left hand travel farther along the hip.

● Place your right leg back and your left leg forward. Use your body weight and strong, straight (but not locked) arms to slide your hands in a deep, slow effleurage stroke up your partner's lower leg.

● Release the pressure as your hands slide over the back of the knee. As you reach the "hamstrings" on the back of the thigh, you may need to adjust your position slightly so that you are not stretching awkwardly.

● Still using your body weight for pressure, circle the upper (left) hand around your partner's hip.

▶ **straight, strong arms** ▶ ▶ **slow, steady pressure** ▶

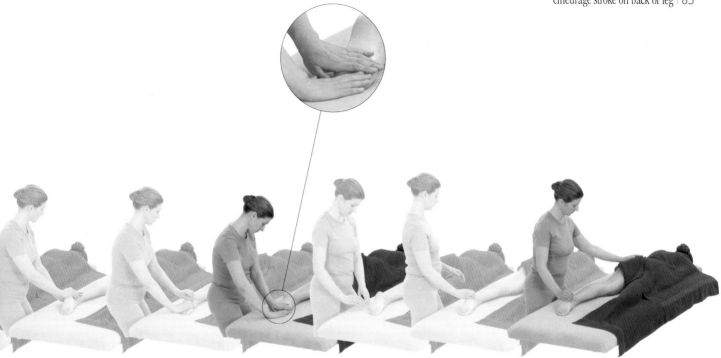

● Without stopping, begin the downward stretch, working with one hand on either side of the leg. Take this opportunity to give the leg a gentle stretch and pull. This helps to give the hip joint a slight release.

● Continue the stretch over the heel and down the foot, bringing your hands right out to the end of the toes.

● The leg massage can now be completed with a hold, by placing your left hand on the left hip and your right hand on the heel. Hold for 5 seconds, and then release and cover the leg.

● Repeat the full back of leg massage on the other leg; then move to the feet and place your hands on the soles of the feet in a connecting hold for 10 seconds. Ask your partner to turn over and adjust the towel as she does so.

▶ **lighter pressure**   ▶   **connecting hold**   ❚❚ ▶   ■

neck stretch

This soothing and releasing neck stretch, which also includes a
shoulder stretch, should not be carried out on anyone suffering
from chronic or degenerative neck problems.

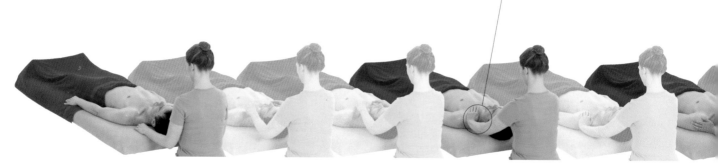

● Position yourself behind your
partner's head and take a moment
to center yourself.

● Let your hands come to rest on
your partner at the points where the
neck meets the shoulders.

● Leaning your body weight through
straight arms, allow your hands to sink
into the shoulder muscle; then begin
a slow, deep slide and stretch down
your partner's shoulders.

● When your hands reach the outer
shoulders, rotate them around the
shoulders and then slide them up to
the base of the neck.

remember posture ▶ **use body weight** ▶

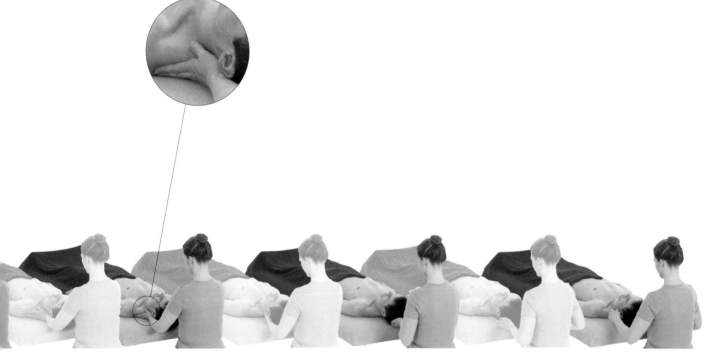

● With one hand above the other, embracing the neck, start a slow, slightly squeezing action to stretch the neck gently. Always make sure that the pressure is on the sides of the neck and not on the spine itself.

● Continue the slow firm, neck stretch.

● Keep the stretch going as your hands slide underneath the head and ease their way out.

● Release your hands to return to their original position on top of the shoulders. This stroke can be repeated two to three times.

slow stretch ▶ ▶ ▶ repeat ⏸ ▶

stretching the pectorals

The strong pectoral muscles lie to either side of the upper
breastbone (sternum) and attach on to the upper arm (humerus).
When these muscles become contracted, the movement of the
arms can become restricted, creating rounded shoulders. This
stroke helps to stretch and release any contraction.

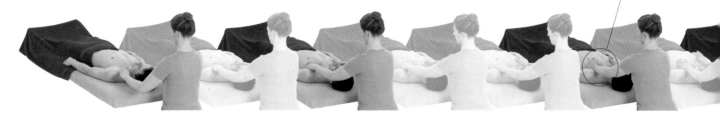

● Still standing behind your partner's
head, take a moment to focus. Rest
your hands on the shoulders.

● Bunch your hands into "soft"
knuckles, placing them just under the
collarbone (clavicle).

● Lean your body weight into your
hands, allowing the soft knuckles to
sink into the muscle tissue of the
upper pectorals. Begin a slow stretch
downward and outward, imagining the
muscles lengthening as you go.

● Repeat this stroke until you feel
that your partner's muscles have
begun to lengthen and relax.

▶ **remember posture** **soft knuckles** ▶ **use body weight** ▶ **straight arms** ▶

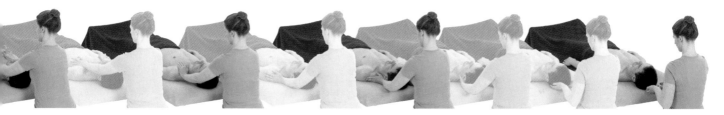

● Working from the same position, this time use the heels of your hands. Start from under the collarbone, stretching downward and outward.

● To complete the stroke, bring your hands back to the tops of the shoulders; then slide and stretch the tops of the shoulders downward and outward.

● Repeat this stroke two or three times. Encourage feedback from your partner to assess the treatment.

● Rotate around and to the back of the shoulders, bringing the stroke up behind the neck. Take your hands underneath the head and then slowly ease them out.

use heels of hands

head and scalp friction massage

The head and scalp massage can be a blissful experience as it helps to discharge released tension from the chest, shoulders, and neck, and to release tight scalp muscles caused by stress, anxiety, and an overworked mind. A head massage also relaxes the hundreds of thousands of muscles that surround all the hairs and follicles on the scalp, bringing blood and nutrients to the area.

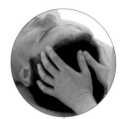

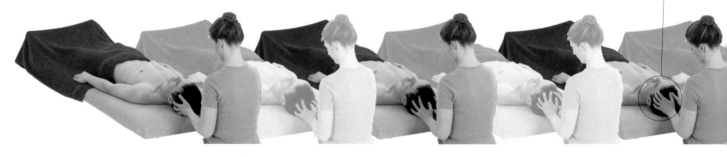

● From the top of the head in the last sequence, bring your hands down to either side of the head, just under the base of the skull.

● Keeping your fingers strong, begin to massage your partner's scalp firmly with this friction stroke.

● The success of this stroke depends on moving the surface skin of the scalp over the bone, using the pads of your fingers and thumbs rather than simply sliding your fingers over the surface of the scalp.

● Gradually start working up the sides of the head. See if you can feel or sense different areas and pockets of tension on the scalp.

▶ **strong fingers** ▶ **massage scalp** ▶ **deep friction circles** ▶

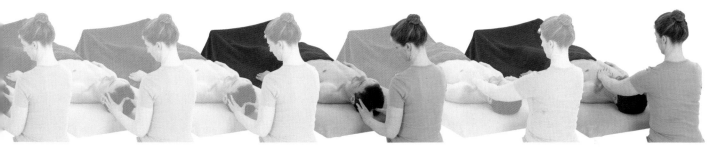

● When your hands reach the top of the head, place your thumbs where the hairline begins.

● Using small, but deep, friction circles, begin to work in a line down the center of the scalp.

● Continue working this friction stroke firmly until you reach the crown of the head; then place your hands on the upper chest in a hold for five seconds to complete the sequence.

● If you are not including a face massage (starting on page 112), place the palms of your hands lightly over the eyes in order to acknowledge the face within the whole body massage.

effleurage up arm

Our arms work for us ceaselessly, carrying, lifting, holding, and supporting, so they respond well to giving up all activity for a time and allowing the "work" to be done by another!

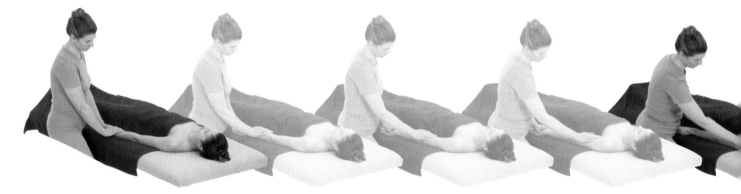

● Oil your hands, and then stand on your partner's left side with your right leg forward and your left leg back. Hold your partner's hand with your left hand to anchor the arm.

● Place the palm of your right hand across the forearm just above the wrist, with your fingers facing toward your partner's body.

● Keeping a straight, strong arm and firm stance, lean your body weight forward into the stroke and begin the slow effleurage slide up the forearm, oiling the arm as you go.

● Let your right hand continue the slow, deep effleurage slide all the way up to the shoulder. Work around the shoulder, rotating the hand in a clockwise direction.

● Your right hand should encompass the contours of the arm while your left hand holds the arm in place. This prevents your partner's shoulder from moving up the couch.

● As the right hand reaches the top of the upper arm, bring the left hand up to the inside of the arm. Use both hands to begin a downward, very gentle stretch and slide.

● Continue the stretch-and-pull action, which gives a gentle joint release to shoulder, elbow, and wrist, taking the stroke out to the end of the hand and fingers.

● Relax your hold as you prepare to move on to massaging the hand and fingers in the next sequence.

effleurage ▶ **light, downward pressure** ▶ ▶ ▶

massaging hands and fingers

Because of the constant application of the hands and fingers in our daily lives, a hand massage is a very pleasant experience. It provides a real release of tension from the muscles, ligaments, tendons, and joints, leaving the hands feeling relaxed and revived.

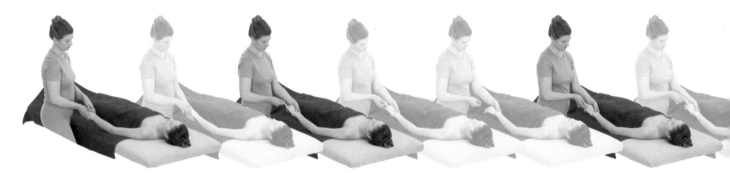

● Still holding your partner's left hand with the palm facing downward, use your fingers and thumbs to stretch, squeeze, and massage the hand, working down from the wrist at ½in (1cm) intervals.

● Work small friction circles with the pads of your thumbs on the top of the hand while your fingers squeeze and stretch. Continue this stroke until you reach the fingers.

● Hold and support the hand with your left hand, while your right hand performs the finger massage. Starting with the little finger, stretch and twist it between your finger and thumb, paying attention to the joints.

● After a final, gentle stretch, release the finger. Move on to the adjacent ring finger and carry out the same massaging, squeezing, and stretching action before pulling and releasing it.

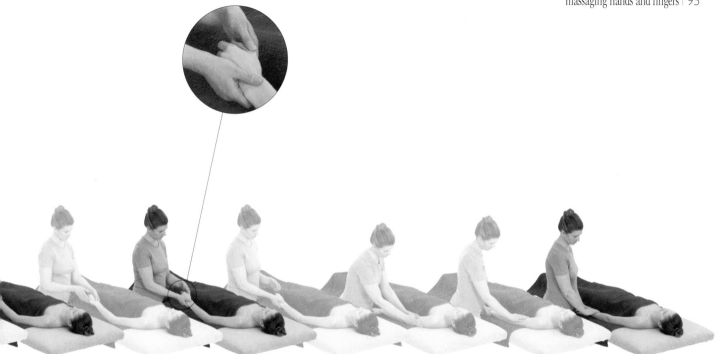

● Take hold of the middle finger, encompassing it with your whole hand. Stretch, massage, and gently pull with your finger and thumb, and spend time on the joints. Release the finger.

● Repeat the massage on the index finger, using the same action as before. Release and move on to the thumb.

● To massage the thumb, transfer your partner's hand to your right hand for support and hold the thumb with your left hand. Massage, squeeze, and gently pull the thumb, spending time on the joints. Place the hand back down on the couch.

● Finish the hand massage with a downward effleurage stretch and clasp your partner's hand between your own in a connecting hold for five seconds.

middle finger ▶ **index finger** ▶ **thumb** ▶ ■

friction stroke over forearm

With so many of us regularly using computers for extended periods, the tendons and muscles of the forearms are subjected to continuous, specific, and constant movements created by intense keyboard activity. The deep friction stroke over the forearm helps to release tension and lengthen the affected muscles and tendons of this area.

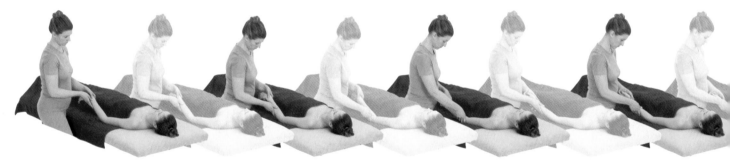

● Pick up your partner's left forearm and turn it to face palm down. Support the hand with your left hand. As the friction stroke works better with just a small amount of oil there should be no need to re-oil the arm at this point.

● Place the fingers of your right hand under the wrist for support and, with your thumb on top, begin to make deep circles above the wrist.

● Let your thumb sink into the muscle tissue, sliding, stretching, and lengthening the muscles as you work up and around the whole area of the outer forearm.

● Turn over your partner's arm so that you can work on the inner side of the forearm.

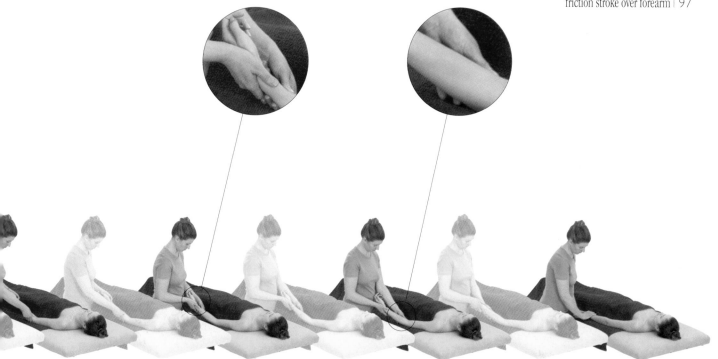

● Pay special attention by working
slowly and deeply into the muscles
close to the elbow since this area can
often be contracted. Gently slide your
hand back to the wrist.

● Now support your partner's wrist
with your right hand and use your left
hand to start deep, circular friction
strokes over the lower inner and
outer forearm, working the areas that
you have not yet covered.

● As you move from the wrist
toward the elbow remember that
with the friction stroke you are sliding
muscle over bone, rather than sliding
your fingers over muscle tissue.

● Slide your hand back to the wrist
and place your partner's hand back on
to the table. Complete the forearm
massage by working an effleurage
stroke over the forearm.

se body weight ▶ ▶ ▶ ▶

soft-knuckle knead on upper arm

This deep, powerful, but gentle stroke is excellent for stretching and lengthening the sometimes contracted muscles (triceps and biceps) and tendons of the upper arm.

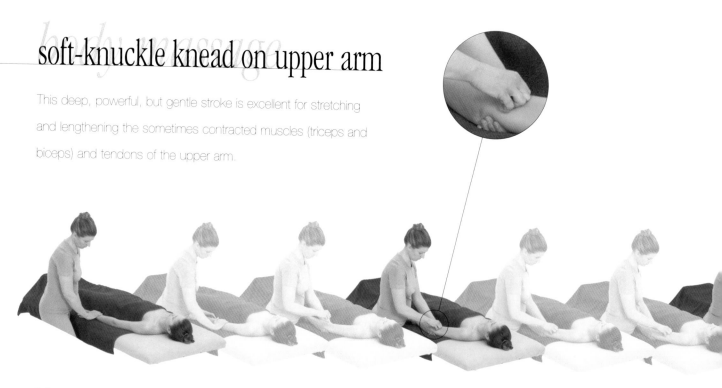

● Starting from the final position on the previous page, hold and support your partner's left hand, facing palm down, with your left hand. Stand with your right leg forward and your left leg back to support this stroke.

● Clasp your partner's arm with your left hand for support and clench your right hand into a loose fist. Keep your arm straight and strong, not letting it collapse at the elbow.

● With the flat and soft part of the knuckle, sink into the muscle tissue of the upper arm, above the elbow, using your body weight for pressure.

● Work into the muscle of the upper arm with deep, circular strokes away from the body. Check that the main pressure is on the outer movement of the circle.

▶   ▶   **use body weight**   ▶   **loose, soft knuckle**

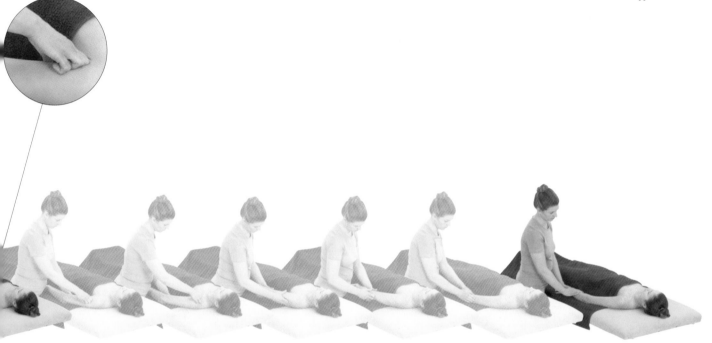

● Circle deeply into the biceps on the inner upper arm and the triceps under the upper arm. Visualize stretching and lengthening all the muscles, thereby creating more space for better functioning joints.

● As you continue to circle up the arm, take the stroke right up to the top of the shoulder where there are many strong connecting tendons and work deeply in this area.

● Take your left hand up to the top of your partner's arm to meet your right hand. Engage both of your hands in gliding down the whole arm, stretching it as you go.

● Two or three effleurage strokes will provide a good completion to the arm massage. Then repeat the whole set of movements (pages 92–99) on the other arm.

circular stretch ▶ ▶ ▶ ■

effleurage up front of leg

This treatment returns the focus and energy to the feet, leaving your partner feeling grounded and centered at the completion of the massage. The opening effleurage stroke has a dual purpose of oiling the front of the leg and stretching, soothing, and preparing the leg for deeper strokes.

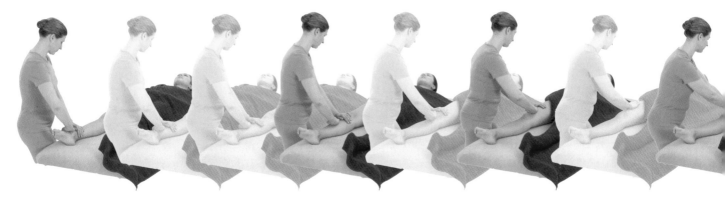

● Uncover your partner's leg and oil your hands. Stand facing the right ankle and, keeping your arms straight, place your right hand across the ankle with fingers pointing left, and your left hand above your right hand in a firm, but not tight, encompassing hold.

● Standing with your left leg forward and your right leg back, lean your body weight through straight, supported arms. Begin to slide your hands slowly over the front of the lower leg toward the knee.

● Use a continuous, controlled motion for this effleurage stroke. At the knee, let your hands stay in contact but lifted sufficiently to slide easily and weightlessly without any pressure over the kneecap (patella).

● Once you have passed the knee, regain the earlier pressure and continue the effleurage stroke, sliding up the upper leg.

remember posture ▶   **less pressure over knee** ▶   **use control** ▶

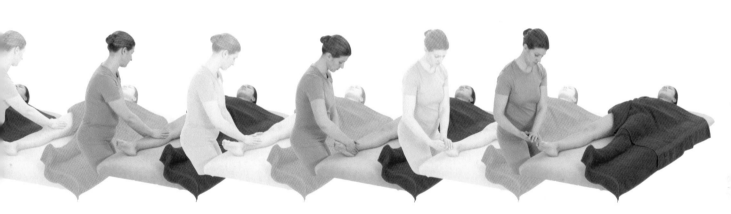

● You will find that your left hand will travel farther up the outer leg while your right hand will stop before reaching the top of the inner thigh.

● As your left hand reaches the top of the outer thigh, rotate it in an outward circle away from you to begin the downward descent.

● When your left and right hands are parallel, encompass your partner's leg, giving it a gentle stretch and pull as both hands descend toward the foot.

● Bring the stroke out the very end of the foot, "sandwiching" it with both hands as you take them right off the ends of the toes. Repeat this stroke two or three times before starting the next sequence.

kneading over front of foot

Once you have followed the techniques explained below in this sequence, you might also like to allow yourself the opportunity of following your intuition as well. Feet can be very expressive and very "needy." See if you can sense and "listen" through your hands to assess what the foot needs!

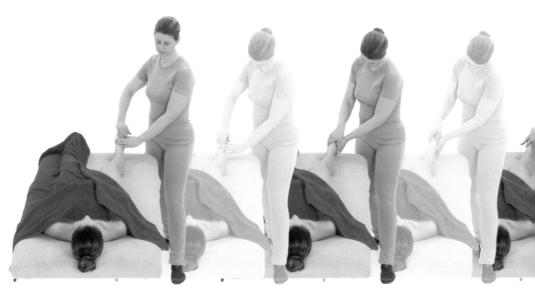

● Oil the foot if it needs lubrication and position yourself so that you can grasp your partner's right foot comfortably with both hands.

● Close your eyes to get the "feel" of your partner's foot; then begin to squeeze and knead the foot with both your hands. Use all of your hand and fingers and include as much of the foot as possible in the massage.

● Continue the motion of squeezing and kneading down the foot until you reach the heel area. Without stopping the movement, start to work your way back to the top of the foot, using the same stroke.

▶   **remember posture**   ▶   **continuous movement**   ▶

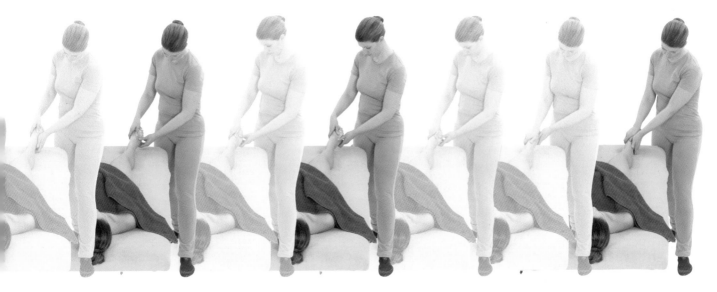

● As you begin the next thumb-friction stroke, encompass and support the foot by placing the fingers of both hands underneath the foot and the thumbs on top.

● Aim to "spread" the tissue on the area above the toes (metatarsal area) as you circle the thumbs away from each other. Continue the movement around the top of the foot, working as deeply as is comfortable for your partner.

● Although it may feel a little strange to massage over the irregular bones of the upper foot (the tarsal bones), it should feel releasing to your partner.

● Remember to take the circles right out to the sides of the foot and under the ankles; then bring the same stroke back to the top of the foot and work your way back to the toes.

▶ **encourage feedback** ▶ ▶ ▶

kneading front lower leg

This stroke provides the opportunity to work deeply on the muscles on either side of the shinbone and into the gastrocnemius and soleus muscles from the front aspect of the lower leg.

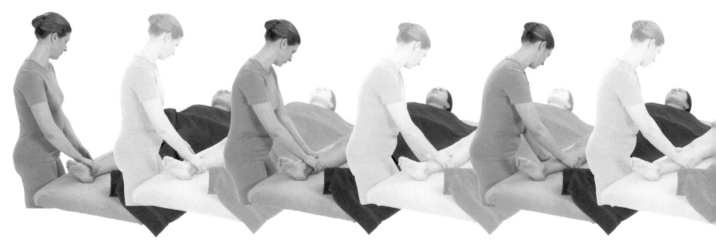

● Stand beside your partner's right ankle, with your left leg forward and right leg back. Place your hands on either side of the shinbone, at the point just above the ankle.

● Use your fingers as supports, placing them under the leg just above the heel. Let the heels of your hands rest on either side of the shinbone.

● With strong, straight arms, lean your body weight into the heels of your hands so that they knead and stretch the muscle tissue in a downward stroke toward your fingers.

● Lean back to release the pressure, slightly lifting your partner's leg. Then, lean forward to bring the heels of your hands down again into the same kneading motion, starting 1in (2.5cm) above the point of the last stroke.

▶   **use body weight**   ▶   **strong, straight arms**   ▶   **lean forward and backward**   ▶

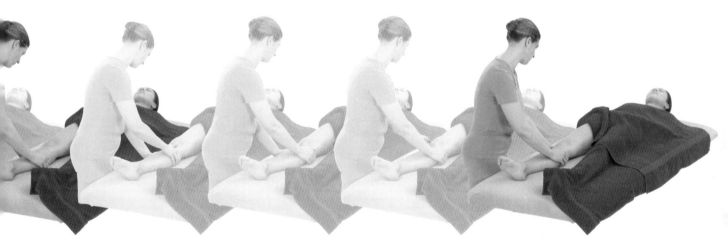

● As you knead and squeeze the muscle tissue of your partner's lower leg, let the stroke become rhythmic with a downward, circular, and then lifting motion.

● Continue with this rhythmic stroke, slowly traveling up the lower leg. As you work, try to detect the stretching effect that is taking place.

● Work the kneading movement until you reach the points below, and either side, of the knee.

● Prepare to slide your hands upward to the point just above the knee, in preparation for the next stage of this stroke to the upper leg.

kneading front upper leg

This kneading stroke, using the heel of the hand, is a continuation of the previous stroke to the lower leg, but works to stretch and release tension in the muscles of the outer thigh (ileo-tibial tract) and the inner thigh (sartorius and adductors).

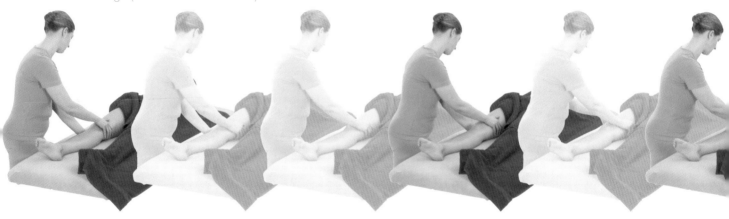

● Continue with the same kneading stroke beside the knee. Spend time on a sensitive pressure point about 1½in (4cm) above the side of the inner knee. In Chinese medicine it relates to the release of tension in the thighs and knees.

● Making sure that you maintain a steady and rhythmic movement, continue to work up the thigh.

● As the inner thigh is a sensitive and private area for your partner, be aware of when you will need to bring your right hand to a respectful stop.

● At the same time let the left hand continue along the outer thigh with a strong downward, kneading motion.

▶   **steady rhythm**   ▶   ▶   **use kneading motion**   ▶

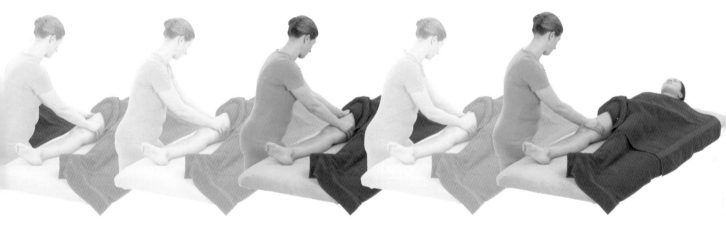

● Use your body weight to create pressure with your left hand as you lift and knead the muscle.

● Continue to work up the thigh until your left hand makes contact with the hip bone.

● Then circle your left hand around the hip bone, moving back and down, until it aligns with your right hand.

● With a slow, firm stretch and pull, slide your hands down to the knee in preparation for the next sequence.

use body weight ▶ ▶ ▶ ▶

wringing from knee to thigh

As the wringing stroke works more effectively over fleshy areas of the body, the thigh and underlying muscles respond well to this stimulating and relaxing stroke.

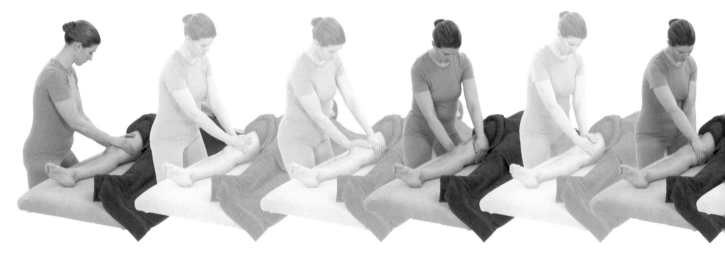

● Turn to face across your partner's body. Although it is unlikely that you will need to re-oil your hands (wringing requires some degree of "grip" to be effective), make sure your partner's skin has enough lubrication.

● Prepare for the stroke by placing both of your hands parallel to each other on the top of your partner's thigh, just above the knee.

● Slide your right hand down to the inner thigh and your left hand outward in a rolling motion. Work them both as far as they can go.

● Bring your hands back to meet each other. Then, without stopping the movement, slide your right hand down and under the inner thigh and your left hand downward and outward.

rhythm ▶ twist ▶ flexible knees ▶

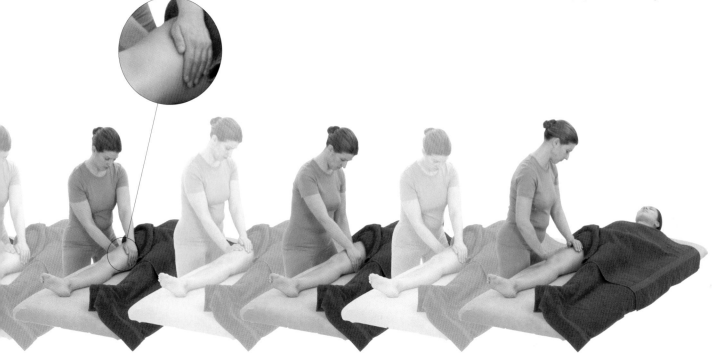

● The secret of this stroke is to achieve a good firm twist and lift to the skin (without causing any pain to your partner) and to establish an energetic, rolling rhythm, such that your body should be almost "dancing."

● Continue to work the wringing stroke along the thigh, each time moving 1 in (2.5cm) above the previous starting point.

● Be aware of the need to maintain a respectful boundary when you reach the top of your partner's inner thigh.

● Bring your hands together at the top of the thigh and take a moment to prepare for the next sequence.

"dancing" body ▶   ▶   ▶   II ▶

front of leg completion

The completion stroke brings the leg massage to a close with a firm downward stretch to the whole of the leg. The hold at the end of the leg massage signals an end to the whole body massage and provides a space for both giver and receiver to reach a point of stillness and integration.

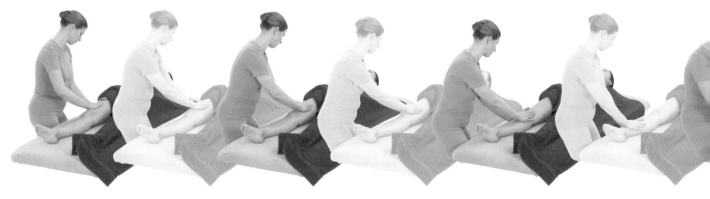

- Turn your body to face your partner, with your upper body facing toward their head.

- Slowly slide your hands away from each other to either side of the leg.

- Using an encompassing stroke combined with a gentle leg stretch, slide your hands down the thigh.

- Keep the stretch going as your hands slide around the knee, gently pulling and stretching as they reach the calf.

gentle downward stretch ▸ use body weight

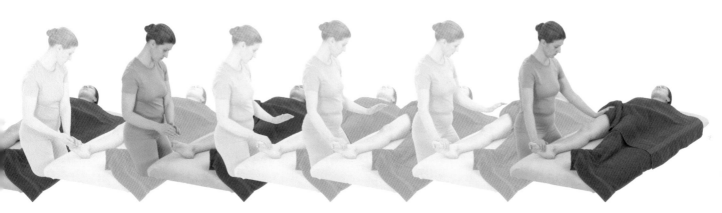

● Work the slide and stretch over the heel, gently squeezing and sliding down the foot. Bring your hands right off and out the end of the toes.

● Place your right hand on top of your partner's foot and your left hand at the hip bone. Make sure you are standing in a position that allows you to reach both points comfortably.

● Close your eyes and visualize the energetic connection between your hands. Let yourself take time to make that connection. You may feel a stillness descend upon you and your partner as this happens.

● Slowly release the contact, cover your partner's leg, and repeat the whole sequence on the other leg. When both legs are massaged and covered, stand at the end of the couch and place your hands on both feet for ten seconds, and then release.

▶ **connect foot and hip**   ▶ **stillness**   ▶   ■

face massage

brow effleurage

The muscles in the forehead respond to anxiety and worry by contracting into furrows and wrinkles. This simple stroke helps to release the tension in this area and, at the same time, relaxes the mind.

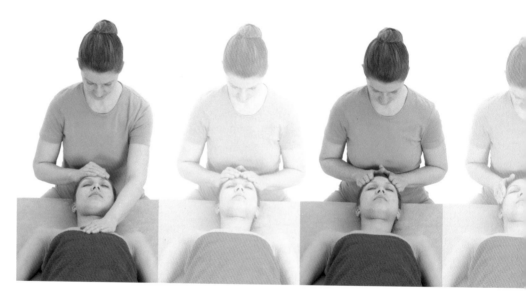

● Sitting comfortably behind your partner's head, start the face and brow massage with a hold. Place your right hand across the forehead and your left hand just below your partner's collarbone (clavicle).

● Hold this position for five seconds to connect and bring about a sense of stillness. Make sure you are not breathing on to your partner's face. Release and lightly oil your hands.

● Place your fingers together at the top of the brow just below the hairline. With a slow, deep stretch, slide your hands away from each other to the sides of the face, keeping the pressure on your fingerpads.

slow, deep stretch

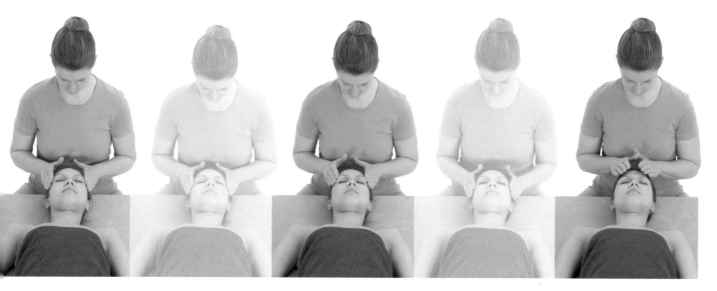

● Feel that you are stretching the muscles under the skin, rather than the skin tissue itself, and that as you release the muscles, so you release the tension within them.

● When the tips of your fingers reach the temples, circle this area slowly and deeply.

● Continue this movement, working two more circles of the temples. It is a common holding area of tension.

● Release the pressure and return your fingers to the starting point on the brow. Repeat the procedure at ½in (1cm) intervals until you reach the area above your partner's eyebrows.

▶ **circle temples** ▶ **breathe freely** ▶ ❚❚ ▶

effleurage over the cheekbones

This stroke stretches the muscle tissue to release any contraction or held tension. Remember to avoid dragging and pulling the skin; instead, massage in an upward and outward movement.

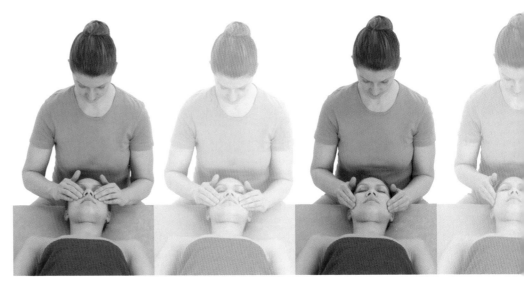

● Lightly re-oil your fingertips and, holding the fingers of each hand together, bring your hands to either side of the nose just beneath the eyes.

● Using an even pressure, contact the muscles beneath the skin and begin to slide your fingers outward over the top of the cheekbones. Notice how this action uses the pads of the fingers rather than the tips.

● Continue to work the stroke, using a sliding movement up and out toward the temples. Bring the hands back to the original position on either side of the face, at the top of the cheekbones.

▶ **use pads of the fingers**　　　**keep fingers together**　▶　　　▶

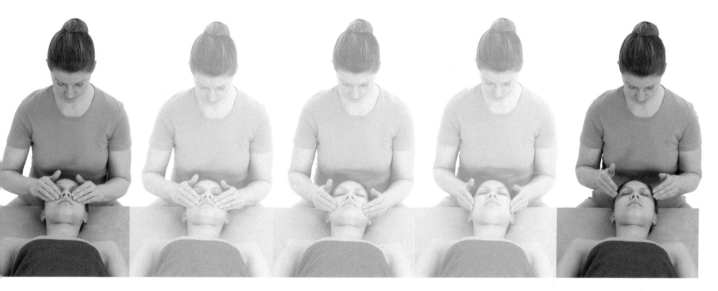

● Repeat the procedure, placing your fingers ¼in (0.5cm) below the starting position.

● Begin the firm, sliding action with the pads of your fingers, making contact with the underlying muscles above the cheekbones.

● Continue working the stroke outward and upward to the temples.

● Repeat the stroke at intervals of ¼in (0.5cm) until your fingers reach the lower ridge of the cheekbones.

deep, slow stretch   **breathe freely**

friction under cheekbones

Working just below the eye and under the cheekbone, this
friction stroke can help blocked sinuses.

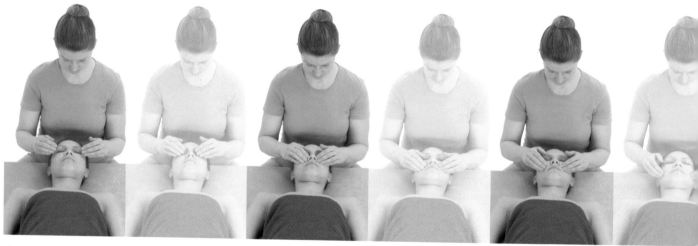

● Hold your fingers together and
slightly curled. Although all of the
fingerpads will be used, the forefinger
will apply most of the pressure.

● Place the pads of your fingers
under the cheekbones close to the
nose. Make sure you do not block
your partner's nostrils.

● Start the massage by working tiny
friction circles under the cheekbones,
pulling the circles toward you.

● For this stroke to be effective, the
friction must be deep and penetrating
with an upward pressure. Remember
that the friction stroke presses tissue
against bone. Check with your partner
for the required comfort level.

▶   ▶ **friction circles**   ▶ **deep, upward pressure**   ▶

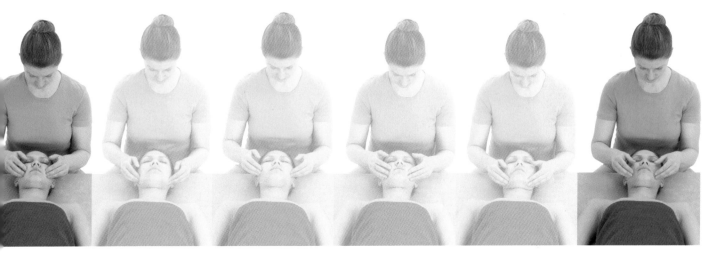

● Using the pads of all your fingers, gradually take the circular friction outward and under the cheekbones.

● As you reach the outer cheekbones your fingers will meet the strong muscle between the upper and lower jaw (the masseter or chewing muscle).

● Begin to work into the masseter muscle, moving gently as it can sometimes be very tight and painful.

● After such a deep stroke, it is best to finish with a little gentle effleurage around the jaw.

breathe freely ▶　　　　▶　gentle movement ▶ repeat ❚❚ ▶

upper lip, chin, and jaw stretch

Expression of strong emotion can be controlled by contracting the upper lip and the muscles of the chin and jaw, hence the phrase "stiff upper lip." This stroke relaxes any tension held in this area.

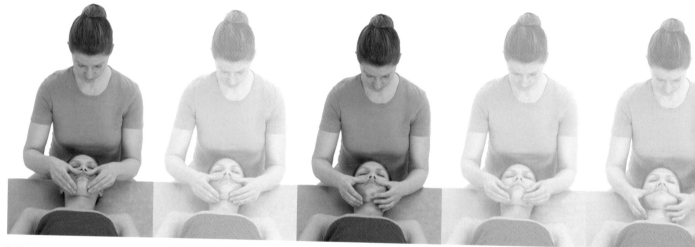

● Holding your hands above the face, bring your thumbs together with your index fingers touching.

● Place your hands on your partner's face so that the pads of the thumbs meet just under the nose, with the fingers meeting underneath the chin.

● With a firm pressure and a slightly upward movement, begin to slide and stretch the upper lip by pulling your thumbs away from each other.

● At the same time, slide your forefingers away from each other, exerting pressure under the chin.

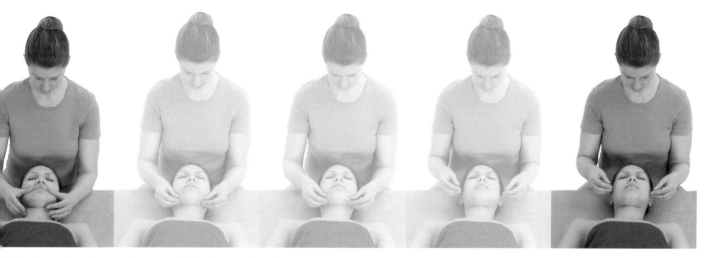

● Continue a slow, deep stretch, taking the thumbs upward and outward away from the upper lip.

● At the same time, slide your forefingers upward, defining the jawline and gently stretching any contracted muscle.

● Slowly and firmly take the stroke out to the junction where the jaw meets the ear.

● Repeat this stroke three times to ensure that any tension in this area has been released.

slow, deep stretch

friction on upper lip and jaw

The effleurage stroke over the upper lip, chin, and jaw (see pages 120–121) prepares this area for the deeper and releasing friction stroke shown in this sequence.

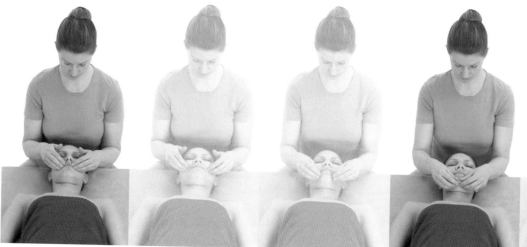

● Place the pads of your forefingers together in the middle of your partner's upper lip to begin the stroke.

● Make tiny and deep friction circles along the upper lip until you reach the cheekbones. Bring the circles toward your body, keeping the pressure on the upward movement so as not to drag the skin tissue downward.

● Gently grasp the chin with your thumbs together and your fingers underneath; then start to make small friction circles. The pressure comes mainly from the thumbs, with the fingers acting as supports.

▶   **deep friction circles**   ▶   **thumb pressure**

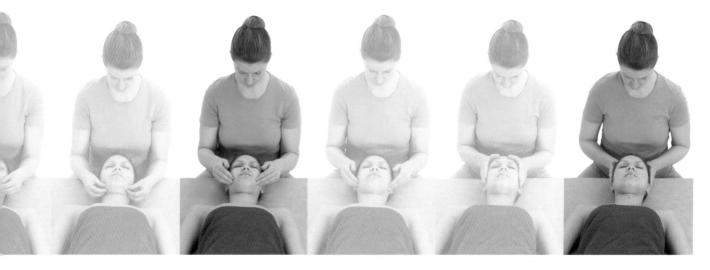

● Using the same stroke, gradually move away from the center of the face and toward the chin.

● Continue to work small but deep friction circles around the outer points of your partner's jaw.

● This will take you into the masseter (or chewing) muscles where you can spend a little time gently working into them with your thumbs or fingers.

● Finish this deep stroke with some gentle and soothing effleurage over the jawline and cheeks. Close with a short five-second hold, placing your hands on either side of the head.

▶   ▶   **deep strokes**   ▶   **gentle effleurage**   ❚❚ ▶

ear massage

Chinese medicine associates the ears with the entire body's energy channels. So your partner may find that a simple ear massage can be an intense (but soothing) experience. For an effective massage, make precise movements and work with intention.

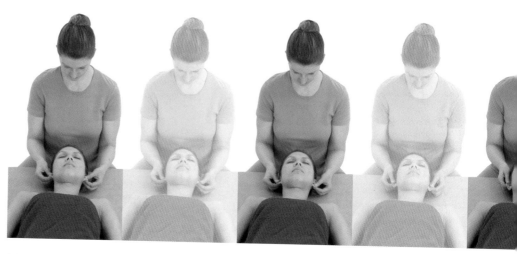

● Lightly oil your fingers and then take hold of your partner's earlobes between your fingers and thumbs.

● Massage the lobes gently but firmly with a rhythmic, circular, outward motion.

● Start to work up the ears, moving over all the undulations using the same circular, outward movement and paying particular attention to the "flap" of the ear.

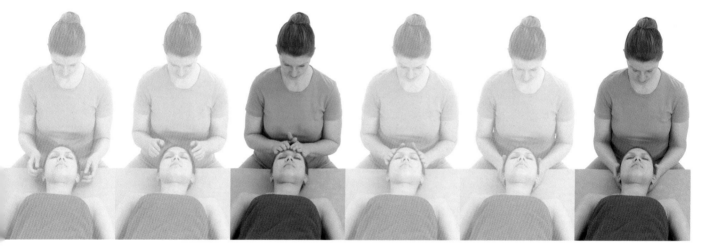

● Continue working thoroughly up to the top of the ear and then start the return journey back down to the lobe.

● Grasping both ears, give them a gentle outward stretch; then release your hands.

● To bring the face massage to a close, place your hands lightly on the top of your partner's head.

● Slide your hands down the sides of the head to complete with a hold. Place your hands on either side of the head for 10 seconds. As an alternative, hold your cupped hands lightly over your partner's eyes for 10 seconds.

work with intention ▶ ▶ ▶ **final hold** ■

index

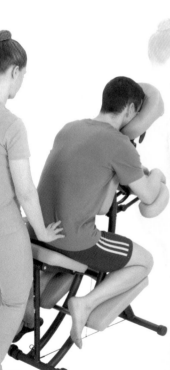
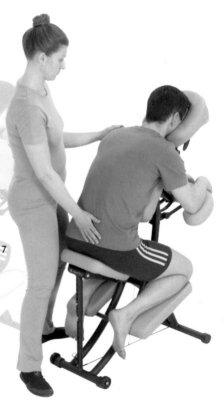

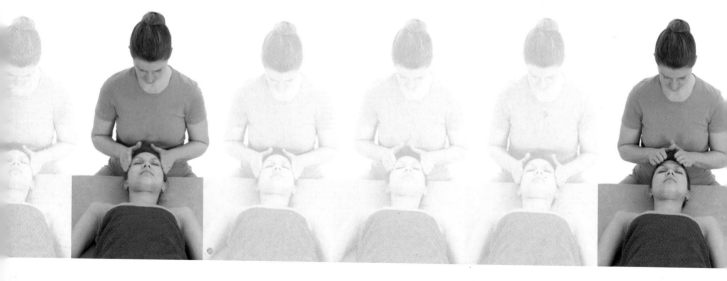